Diabetic
Meal Prep
for
Beginners

Diabetic Meal Prep for Beginners provides the healthiest, tastiest, and quickest meal options to control and conquer your diabetes.

---

4 - WEEK MEAL PLAN

100+ Recipes

Sara Green

Table of Contents

Diabetic Meal Prep for Beginners

Introduction

Nearly half a billion people worldwide endure the struggle of living with diabetes. In many countries, diabetes has become a health epidemic of massive proportions. In the USA alone, over nine percent of the population (roughly 31 million Americans) suffers some form of this disease (Centers for Disease Control and Prevention, 2016). Those suffering from diabetes require specific diets to stay fit and in good health. And so, in this book, I hope to provide a comprehensive guide on how to eat healthily in the easiest way possible for those of us with diabetes. But first, let us explore what diabetes is and how we cope with it.

What Is Diabetes?

Diabetes mellitus, commonly known just as diabetes, is a disease that affects our metabolism. The predominant characteristic of diabetes is an inability to create or utilize insulin, a hormone that moves sugar from our blood cells into the rest of our bodies' cells. This is crucial for us because we rely on that blood sugar to power our body and provide energy. High blood sugar, if left untreated, can lead to serious damage of our eyes, nerves, kidneys, and other major organs. There are two major types of diabetes, type 1 and type 2, with the latter being the most common of the two with over 90 percent of diabetics suffering from it (Centers for Disease Control and Prevention, 2019).

HOW DOES INSULIN WORK?

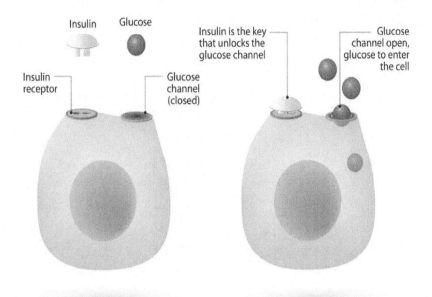

Insulin

Glucose

Insulin receptor

Glucose channel (closed)

Insulin is the key that unlocks the glucose channel

Glucose channel open, glucose to enter the cell

Type 1 diabetes is an autoimmune disease. In cases of type 1 diabetes, the immune system attacks cells in the pancreas responsible for insulin production. Although we are unsure what causes this reaction, many experts believe it is brought upon by a gene deficiency or by viral infections that may trigger the disease.

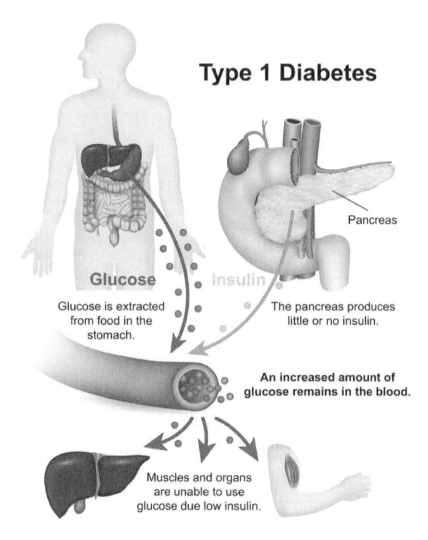

Type 1 Diabetes

Pancreas

Glucose

Insulin

Glucose is extracted from food in the stomach.

The pancreas produces little or no insulin.

An increased amount of glucose remains in the blood.

Muscles and organs are unable to use glucose due low insulin.

Type 2 diabetes is a metabolic disorder, although research suggests it may warrant reclassification as an autoimmune disease as well. People who suffer from type 2 diabetes have a high resistance to insulin or an inability to produce enough insulin. Experts believe that type 2 diabetes is a result of a genetic predisposition in many people, which is further aggravated by obesity and other environmental triggers.

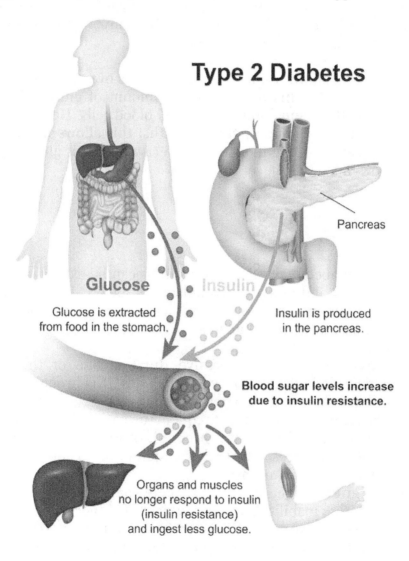

Type 2 Diabetes

Pancreas

Glucose

Insulin

Glucose is extracted from food in the stomach.

Insulin is produced in the pancreas.

Blood sugar levels increase due to insulin resistance.

Organs and muscles no longer respond to insulin (insulin resistance) and ingest less glucose.

Diagnosis

Diabetes diagnosis has come incredibly far in the last few decades. Currently, there are two primary tests for diagnosing diabetes: the fasting plasma glucose (FPG) test and the hemoglobin A1c test.

The FPG test measures your blood sugar levels after an eight-hour fasting period; this helps to show if your body is processing glucose at a healthy rate.

The A1c test shows your blood sugar levels over the last three months. It does this by testing the amount of glucose being carried by the hemoglobin of your red blood cells. Hemoglobin has a lifespan of roughly three months; this allows us to test them to see how long they have been carrying their glucose for and how much they have.

Symptoms

In type 1 diabetes, the list of symptoms can be extensive with both serious and less obvious indicators. Below, I will list the most common symptoms as well as other potential complications of type 1 diabetes:

- **Excessive thirst:** Excessive thirst is one of the less noticeable indicators of type 1 diabetes. It is brought upon by high blood sugar (hyperglycemia).
- **Frequent urination:** Frequent urination is caused by your kidneys failing to process all of the glucose in your blood; this forces your body to attempt to flush out excess glucose through urinating.
- **Fatigue:** Fatigue in type 1 diabetes patients is caused by the body's inability to process glucose for energy.
- **Excessive hunger:** Those suffering from type 1 diabetes often have persistent hunger and increased appetites. This is because the body is desperate for glucose despite its inability to process it without insulin.

- **Cloudy or unclear vision:** Rapid fluctuations in blood sugar levels can lead to cloudy or blurred vision. Those suffering from untreated type 1 diabetes are unable to naturally control their blood sugar levels, making rapid fluctuations a very common occurrence.
- **Rapid weight loss:** Rapid weight loss is probably the most noticeable symptom of type 1 diabetes. As your body starves off glucose, it resorts to breaking down muscle and fat to sustain itself. This can lead to incredibly fast weight loss in type 1 diabetes cases.
- **Ketoacidosis:** Ketoacidosis is a potentially deadly complication of untreated type 1 diabetes. In response to the lack of glucose being fed into your muscles and organs, your body starts breaking down your fat and muscle into an energy source called ketones, which can be burned without the need of insulin. Ketones are usually perfectly fine in normal amounts. But, when your body is starving, it may end up flooding itself with ketones in an attempt to fuel itself; the acidification of your blood that follows this influx of acid molecules may lead to more serious conditions, a coma, or death.

SYMPTOMS OF TYPE 1 DIABETES

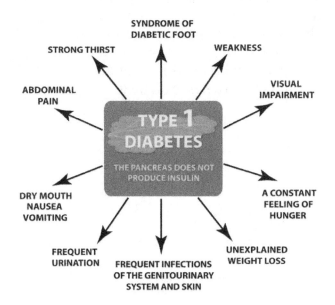

SYNDROME OF DIABETIC FOOT

STRONG THIRST

WEAKNESS

ABDOMINAL PAIN

VISUAL IMPAIRMENT

TYPE 1 DIABETES

THE PANCREAS DOES NOT PRODUCE INSULIN

DRY MOUTH NAUSEA VOMITING

A CONSTANT FEELING OF HUNGER

FREQUENT URINATION

FREQUENT INFECTIONS OF THE GENITOURINARY SYSTEM AND SKIN

UNEXPLAINED WEIGHT LOSS

In cases of type 2 diabetes, the symptoms tend to be slower to develop, and they tend to be mild early on. Some early symptoms mimic type 1 diabetes and may include:

- **Excessive hunger:** Similar to type 1 diabetes, those of us with type 2 diabetes will feel constant hunger. Again, this is brought on by our bodies looking for fuel because of our inability to process glucose.
- **Fatigue and mental fog:** Depending on the severity of the insulin shortage in type 2 sufferers, they may feel physical fatigue and a mental fogginess during their average day.
- **Frequent urination:** Another symptom of both type 1 and 2 diabetes. Frequent urination is simply your body's way of attempting to rid itself of excess glucose.
- **Dry mouth and constant thirst:** It is unclear what causes dry mouth in diabetic sufferers, but it is tightly linked to high blood sugar levels. Constant thirst is brought on not only by a dry mouth but also by the dehydration that frequent urination causes.
- **Itchy skin:** Itching of the skin, especially around the hands and feet, is a sign of polyneuropathy (diabetic nerve damage). As well as being a sign of potential nerve damage, itching can be a sign of high concentrations of cytokines circulating in your bloodstream; these are inflammatory molecules that can lead to itching. Cytokines are signaling proteins and hormonal regulators that are often released in high amounts before nerve damage.

SYMPTOMS OF TYPE 2 DIABETES

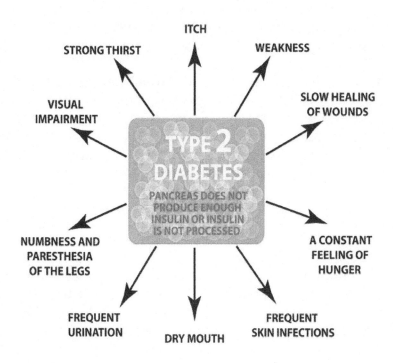

As type 2 diabetes progresses and becomes more serious, the symptoms can become highly uncomfortable and dangerous. Some of these advanced symptoms include:

- **Slow healing of bruises, cuts, and abrasions:** Many people suffering from type 2 diabetes have impaired immune systems due to the lack of energy available to the body. As well as a lack of energy, many diabetics have slowed circulation brought upon by high blood glucose levels. Both of these factors lead to a much slower healing process and far greater risks of infection.
- **Yeast infections:** In women with type 2 diabetes, the chances of yeast infections are far higher than in

non-diabetic women. This is due to high blood sugar levels and a lowered immune system response.

- **Neuropathy or numbness:** Long-term high blood sugar levels can lead to severe nerve damage in adults with diabetes. It is believed around 70 percent of people with type 2 diabetes have some form of neuropathy (Hoskins, 2020). Diabetic neuropathy is characterized by a numbness in the extremities, specifically around the feet and fingers.
- **Dark skin patches (acanthosis nigricans):** Some people with type 2 diabetes may have far above normal levels of insulin in their blood, as their body is unable to utilize it due to insulin resistance. This increase of insulin in the bloodstream can lead to some skin cells over reproducing and cause dark patches to form on the skin.

Complications

Severe complications of diabetes can be debilitating and deadly. Both type 1 and type 2 diabetes can lead to serious neurological, cardiovascular, and optical conditions. *Some of the most common complications of advanced diabetes are as follows:*

- **Heart attacks:** Diabetes is directly linked to a higher rate of heart attacks in adults. High blood glucose levels damage the cells and nerves around the heart and blood vessels over time, which can cause a plethora of heart diseases to form.
- **Cataracts:** People with diabetes have a nearly 60 percent greater chance of developing cataracts later in life if their diabetes is left unchecked (Diabetes.co.uk, 2019a). Doctors are unsure of the exact reason for cataracts forming at a higher rate in diabetes patients, but many believe it has to do with the lower amounts of glucose available to the cells powering our eyes.
- **Peripheral artery disease (PAD):** This is a very common complication of diabetes in which the blood vessels in the legs become blocked or narrowed due to fat

16

deposits. This causes decreased blood flow, which leads to serious issues in the lower legs, often resulting in amputation.

- **Diabetic nephropathy:** Diabetic nephropathy happens when high levels of blood glucose damage parts of your kidneys, which is responsible for filtering blood. This causes your kidneys to develop chronic kidney diseases and break down over time, leading to failure.

- **Glaucoma:** Diabetes can cause glaucoma in sufferers due to high blood sugar levels and this directly damages blood vessels in the eyes. When your body attempts to repair these vessels, it may cause glaucoma on the iris where the damage was caused.

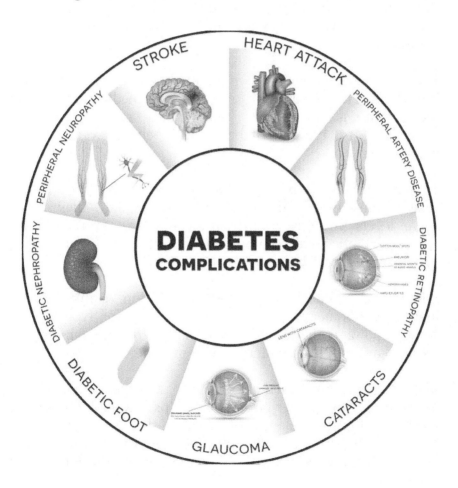

Treatment

Treatments for diabetes vary depending on the type, number, and severity of complications and health of the patient overall. Luckily, diabetes has been long studied by the medical community and, therefore, there is an abundance of resources and treatments available.

For type 1 diabetes, insulin supplements are essential. Type 1 diabetics rely on daily insulin injections; some prefer a costlier but easier-to-use insulin pump. Insulin needs in type 1 diabetics will vary throughout the day as they eat and exercise. This means many type 1 diabetics will regularly test their blood sugar levels to assess whether their insulin needs are being met.

Some type 1 diabetics develop insulin resistance after years of injections. This means that oral diabetes medication such as metformin is becoming increasingly more commonly prescribed to type 1 diabetics to help prevent insulin resistance.

Type 2 diabetes can be controlled without medication in some cases. Many type 2 diabetics can self-regulate their blood sugar levels through careful eating and light exercise. Most type 2 diabetics are recommended to stay on low-fat diets, which are high in fiber and healthy carbs.

Some type 2 diabetics do need medication. Unlike type 1, insulin is not nearly as commonly needed for type 2. But, some type 2 diabetics do need insulin to supplement the reduced amount their pancreas may provide.

The most common medication given to type 2 diabetics is metformin. This prescription drug helps lower blood glucose levels and improve insulin sensitivity. Other drugs prescribed to type 2 diabetics include sulfonylureas, thiazolidinediones, and meglitinides, which all help increase insulin production or sensitivity.

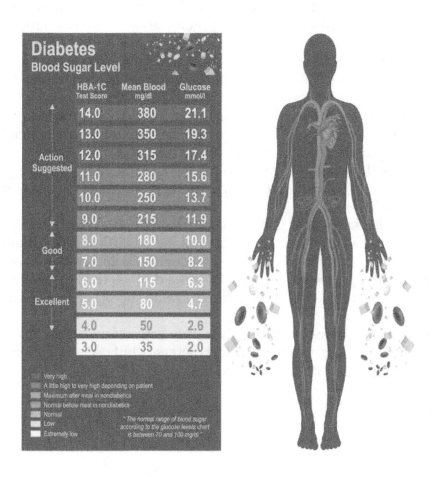

Diabetes
Blood Sugar Level

	HBA-1C Test Score	Mean Blood mg/dl	Glucose mmol/l
	14.0	380	21.1
	13.0	350	19.3
Action Suggested	12.0	315	17.4
	11.0	280	15.6
	10.0	250	13.7
	9.0	215	11.9
Good	8.0	180	10.0
	7.0	150	8.2
	6.0	115	6.3
Excellent	5.0	80	4.7
	4.0	50	2.6
	3.0	35	2.0

Very high
A little high to very high depending on patient
Maximum after meal in nondiabetics
Normal before meal in nondiabetics
Normal
Low
Extremely low

" The normal range of blood sugar according to the glucose levels chart is between 70 and 100 mg/dl "

10 Tips to Control Diabetes

- **Eat less salt:** Salt can increase your chances of having high blood pressure, which leads to increased chances of heart disease and stroke.
- **Replace sugar:** Replace sugar with zero calorie sweeteners. Cutting out sugar gives you much more control over your blood sugar levels.
- **Cut out alcohol:** Alcohol tends to be high in calories, and if drunk on an empty stomach with insulin medication, it can cause drastic drops in blood sugar.

- **Be physically active:** Physical activity lowers your risk of cardiovascular issues and increases your body's natural glucose burn rate.
- **Avoid saturated fats:** Saturated fats like butter and pastries can lead to high cholesterol and blood circulation issues.
- **Use canola or olive oil:** If you need to use oil in your cooking, use canola or olive oil. Both are high in beneficial fatty acids and monounsaturated fat.
- **Drink water:** Water is by far the healthiest drink you can have. Drinking water helps to regulate blood sugar and insulin levels.
- **Make sure you get enough vitamin D:** Vitamin D is a crucial vitamin for controlling blood sugar levels. Eat food high in this vitamin or ask your doctor about supplements.
- **Avoid processed food:** Processed foods tend to be high in vegetable oils, salt, refined grains, or other unhealthy additives.
- **Drink coffee and tea:** Not only are coffee and tea great hunger suppressants for dieters, but they contain important antioxidants that help with protecting cells.

Chapter 1: The Role of Food

The role of food in diabetes care is crucial. Finding a balance in the right combination of carbs, fats, proteins, fiber, vitamins, and minerals is important in maintaining a healthy diet and lifestyle. Getting this balance right is a challenge many diabetics struggle with, but with the right diet and meal plan, it can be easily achieved.

For decades, dietitians, nutritionists, doctors, and scientists have been arguing over the ideal mix of nutrients that are needed for optimum diabetic health. Only in the past few years, however, have we started to get a clearer picture of the exact type of diet we need to follow.

When breaking down our food groups, we end up with what are referred to as the three macro-nutrients. These are proteins, carbohydrates, and fats. The importance of these foods is that they make up our primary sources of energy. Fats and proteins provide much-needed amino acids for building cells and slow burning glucose, whilst carbohydrates help build up our energy reserves and act as a fast-acting source of glucose energy.

The Effects of Certain Food on Diabetes

Certain foods have drastic impacts on the health of diabetics, both in good and bad respects. With the balance of blood sugar being as important as it is for diabetics, various foods, which help regulate blood sugar or slow down the digestion of glucose-heavy foods, can be a key part of diabetic dieting. On the contrary, some foods may be dangerously high in sugars and high glucose carbs, which can terribly upset the balance of blood sugar in some people.

Before we get into what foods are good and which should be avoided, it is wise to remember that too much of anything can be bad for you. Too much protein or fat can lead to high blood sugar; the same as that can happen if you consume too many carbs. How much you need to be eating depends on your age, weight, gender, and level of activity. Typically, a diet for diabetics looking to lose weight is around 1,500-1,800 calories per day (Norman, 2019).

The meal plan later in this book is a perfect example of a balanced diabetic diet. The majority of your daily calories come from healthy carbs and proteins, with a minority made up of sugar.

THE GLUCOSE LEVEL

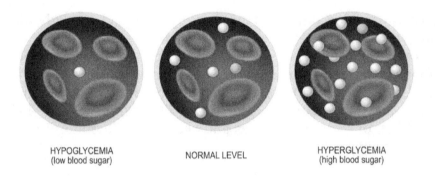

HYPOGLYCEMIA
(low blood sugar)

NORMAL LEVEL

HYPERGLYCEMIA
(high blood sugar)

Which Food Hinders

Out of the three macronutrients, we rely on, carbohydrates have the greatest impact on our blood sugar levels. This is because carbs are broken down into glucose incredibly quickly and efficiently by our bodies. Therefore, any diabetic diet should look to limit and closely watch the amount of carbs they consume.

Carbs can be split into starches, sugars, and fibers. Fiber is the only carb we won't necessarily look to remove as it digests in a way that doesn't raise our blood sugar. Fiber often accompanies starch and sugar in foods, so when we calculate the carb content of a meal, we calculate the net carb count rather than the total carb count. An example of that would be a bowl of vegetables containing 15 grams of carbs in total but four grams of that being fiber. Therefore, the net carbs would only be 11 grams.

Foods that should be avoided in most diabetic diets are as follows:

- **Sugary drinks:** Avoid drinks such as soda, sweetened iced tea, lemonade, fruit juices, beer, and sweet wines. Researchers have shown that our brains don't process liquid in the same way they process solid food. When we drink calories, we don't eat less later to compensate. This can lead to consistently high glucose levels.
- **White bread, pasta, and rice:** High-carb, processed foods contain very little fiber, which causes them to digest very quickly, flooding the bloodstream with glucose and causing spikes in blood sugar levels.
- **Honey, syrup, and agave nectar:** These natural sugars contain even more carbs per gram than normal white sugar.
- **Sweetened cereals and mueslis:** Breakfast cereals contain very high amounts of processed carbs with very low amounts of protein. This not only leads to spikes in blood sugar but without protein's satiating properties, you will start feeling hungry again in no time.
- **Flavored yogurt:** Flavored yogurts are typically packed with sugars and carbs, whether from sweeteners, fruit nectars, or fruit chunks. Plain, sugar-free yogurts are far healthier for your gut health and blood sugar levels.
- **Dried fruit:** Unfortunately, even some food we think of as healthy can upset our blood sugar balance. Dried fruits have an even higher concentration of sugar than fresh fruit. Raisins have been shown to have nearly three times as much sugar as fresh grapes.
- **French fries:** Potatoes themselves are less than ideal for a diabetic diet. But, once we peel and fry them, they

become even more hazardous. Fried potatoes not only contain high amounts of carbs but also large amounts of inflammatory compounds such as aldehydes. These compounds can impact cardiovascular health and bring upon heart disease in high risk diabetic patients.

- **Candy, cookies, and ice cream:** This one may seem obvious but many people still indulge a bit too much in these guilty pleasures. Candy, cookies, ice cream, and any other high sugar treats can send blood sugar spiking up very high. These types of food digest very quickly and flood your system with glucose faster than your body can handle.

Which Food Helps

There is a plethora of foods that help with regulating and controlling our blood sugar levels. Luckily, these foods are not only tasty, but readily available and easy to cook with.

Typically, we'll look to replace the carbs in a non-diabetic diet with healthy fats, proteins, and high-fiber carbs to turn it into a diabetic-friendly diet. Many experts still debate over whether the space left by carbs should be filled more by protein or by fat, but one thing they all agree on is that either way is healthier than a carb-heavy diet.

Foods that help diabetes control their blood sugar levels are as follows:

- Leafy green vegetables: Leafy greens are very low in calories and yet extremely nutritious. Vegetables like spinach, kale, and broccoli are fantastic sources of vitamins and minerals. Green vegetables have also been shown to be high in natural antioxidants, which promote better heart and eye health.

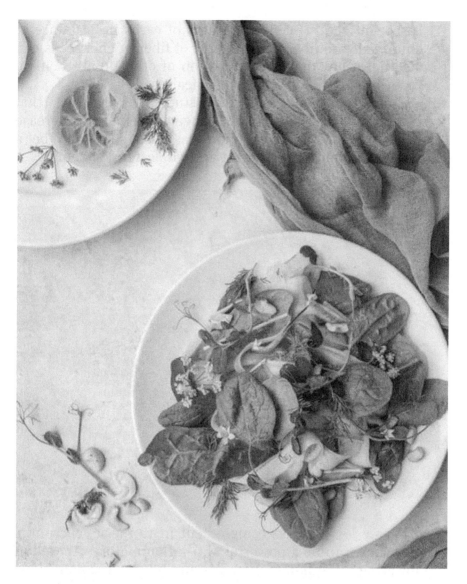

- **Fatty fish:** Fish like sardines, salmon, herring, mackerel, and anchovies are amazing sources of fatty acids that promote heart health. Consuming these fats regularly is especially important for diabetics who are at great risk of cardiovascular disease. These fish are also a great source of protein, which makes us feel full and provides plenty of energy to replace the sugar we have cut.
- **Chia seeds:** These seeds make a fantastic ingredient and snack for diabetics. Chia seeds contain nearly no sugary

carbs; in fact, 11 of the 12 grams of carbs in an ounce of chia seeds are fiber. The amount of fiber in chia seeds can also help slow down the digestion of other foods, helping to lower your blood sugar after meals.

- Cinnamon: Multiple clinical studies have shown that cinnamon can lower blood sugar levels and increase insulin sensitivity. Cinnamon has also shown to be a strong antioxidant with great anti-cholesterol benefits.

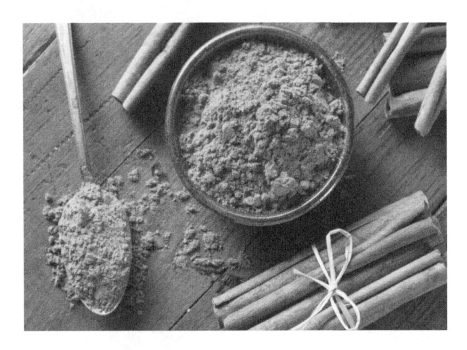

- Turmeric: The active ingredient in turmeric, curcumin, has shown to be a powerful anti-inflammatory. As well as lowering cell inflammation, curcumin helps regulate blood sugar levels, protect against heart disease, and benefit kidney health.
- Eggs: Not only are eggs incredibly satiating, but they also provide some fantastic health benefits many people overlook. These fantastic little ovals have powerful anti-inflammatories and antioxidants that help improve cardiovascular function, improve insulin sensitivity, cut down on cholesterol, and promote good eye health.
- Broccoli: Because broccoli is so awesome, I've decided to give it its own bullet point even though it is still part of the

leafy greens you read about above. This is one of the healthiest vegetables easily available to us. A cup of cooked broccoli contains only 50 calories and 6 grams of carbs. Broccoli is packed with vitamin C, magnesium, and calcium, along with plenty of other great vitamins and minerals.

- **Nuts:** All nuts are high in fiber and low in sugary carbs, so they make a perfect snack for diabetics. Per ounce serving, Brazil nuts, hazelnuts, macadamia, pecan, and walnuts have the lowest amount of digestible sugary carbs. As well as being very satiating, nuts have also shown to have properties that lower blood sugar and reduce inflammation.

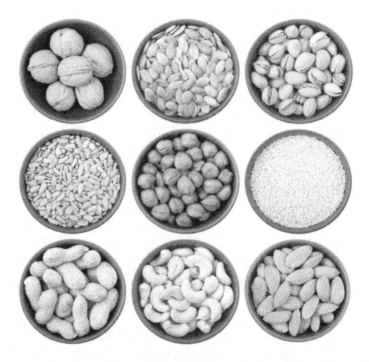

- **Extra-virgin olive oil:** A fantastic cooking ingredient and salad dressing, but also the only fat has proven to lower risks of heart disease. Olive oil has shown to lower cholesterol levels and help with cardiovascular health. Olive oil also contains polyphenols, an antioxidant that protects blood vessels and lowers inflammation.

What is the glycemic index?

The glycemic index (GI) indicates the ability of a food to raise blood sugar, expressed as a percentage of a reference food (glucose or white bread). A high GI, therefore, leads to greater growth in blood sugar, with the same carbohydrate content.

Which foods have the highest glycemic index?

Among the foods with a high GI is white bread, which increases blood sugar more than many other foods. Potatoes also have a high index. Among the meals, semolina pasta has a lower GI than polished rice (better choose brown rice), especially if it is not overcooked. Cooking food influences the GI value and is a good recommendation, therefore, to prefer pasta and rice "al dente".

Which foods have the lowest glycemic index?

Legumes, skim milk, yogurt, tomatoes, and fresh fruit. To avoid glycemic peaks, the amount of dietary fiber we take with our diet is also very important. It is a particular type of carbohydrate that is not digested, and which slows down the absorption of sugars and fats in the intestine.

Avoiding too many carbohydrates is a good rule of thumb, not only for those with diabetes but for anyone who wants to keep fit by keeping their blood sugar checked. For this, it is useful to consider the glycemic index of foods.

Glycemic index indicates how foods affect blood sugar and insulin. The lower a food's glycemic index or glycemic load, the lesser it affects blood sugar and insulin levels. Here are over 100 common foods with glycemic index and glycemic load.

The glycemic index gives you an idea of how quickly your body converts the carbohydrates of a food into glucose 2 foods with the same amount of carbohydrates that can have different glycemic index numbers. The smaller the number, the lesser the impact of food on blood sugar.

Glycemic Index Chart

Low 55 or Less		Medium 56-69		High 70 or Higher	
Asparagus	15	Wild Rice	57	Whole Wheat	71
Broccoli	15	Sweet Potatoes	69	Muesli Bread	80
Celery	15	Muesli	66	Baked Potatoes	85
Cucumber	15	Cous Cous	65	Puffed wheat	80
Lettuce	15	Mango	56	Graham Crackers	74
Peppers	15	Pineapple	66	White Bread	76
Spinach	15	Grapes,average	59	Watermelon	72
Tomatoes	15	Ice Cream	61	Doughnut	78
Chickpeas	33	Black-Eyed Beans	69	Jelly Beans	80
Cooked Carrots	39	Pancakes	67	Pretzels	83
Grapefruit	25	Oatmeal	56	Rice Cakes	82
Apple	38	Banana	60	Pumpkin	76
Peach	42	Beets	64	French Fries	75
Orange	44	Raisins	62	Instant Oatmeal	83
Mushrooms	10	Cheese Pizza	67	White Rice	89
Low-Fat Yogurt	14	Wheat Thins	68	Fruit Rollup	99
Plain Yogurt	14	Pita Bread	68	Baguette (white)	96
Whole Milk	27	Taco Shells	65	Waffels	76
Soy Milk	30	Cantaloupe	65	Soda Crakers	74
Skim Milk	32				
Chocolate Milk	35	**Beverages**			
Fruit Yogurt	36				
Peanuts	21	Coca Cola		63	
Beans, Dried	40	Fanta		68	
Lentils	41	Lucozade		95	
Kidney Beans	41	Apple Juice		44	
Split Peas	45	Cranberry Juice Cocktail		68	
Lima Beans	46	Gatorade		78	
Rice Bran	27	Orange Juice		50	
Bran Cereal	42	Tomato Juice		38	
Spaghetti	42	Red Wine		15	
Corn, sweet	54	Beer		15	

Chapter 2: What Is Meal Prep?

Meal prep has become a necessity in this day and age. Many of us work hard and just don't have the energy to spend an hour cooking dinner when we get home. We'd much rather just grab something easy to eat and relax. This is where meal preparation enters into our lives. Instead of getting home from work every day, preparing ingredients, cooking, and cleaning up, we'll prepare some or all of our food on one day.

Meal prepping is beneficial in so many ways and it's criminal that more people don't use it to its full extent. We save so much money by buying our own ingredients and cooking in bulk at home. Takeaways or meal delivery services are expensive, and meal prep will be noticeably cheaper. And, we'll be eating such healthier meals by avoiding processed and fried foods!

As a diabetic, keeping track of when you eat and what you eat can be very important towards your general health. By following a diabetic meal prep plan, you can track ahead of time what you're going to be eating, and when you'll be eating it. This is especially useful for busy diabetics who don't have the time to track calories during the work day.

Where to Start :

Starting with meal prep is very simple; your best friends will be reusable, airtight food storage containers. We want airtight containers to keep out bacteria and keep our food fresh. Containers with removable dividers are fantastic, as we can split up portions or parts of our meal that we don't want to mix together.

Once you've got your containers, you need to decide what type of meal prep you want to do. Meal prep is very flexible, so if you have specific dietary needs, are on a budget, or really short on time, you always have an option. The most popular forms of meal prep include:

- **Batch cooking:** Cooking large batches of particular foods such as hotpots, soups, then breaking the batches up into meal portions, which can be frozen for meals over the coming weeks. This is a very popular method for easy-to-prepare hot dinners and lunches.

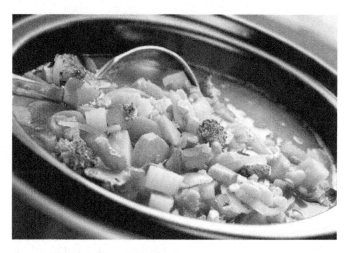

- **Make-ahead meals:** These are full meals of mains and sides that are prepared in advance and refrigerated for dinners over the coming week. Typically, these include ingredients we don't want to freeze and would rather eat within a few days of prep.

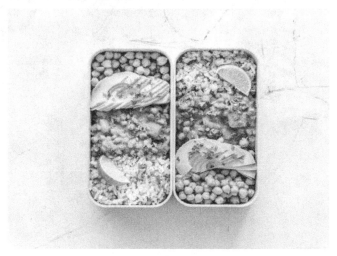

- **Individual meal portions:** Different from make-ahead meals in that these are small portions of fresh foods, like chicken salads, stir fries, or wraps. These are perfect for quick grab-and-go lunches and don't necessarily need to be heated up beforehand.

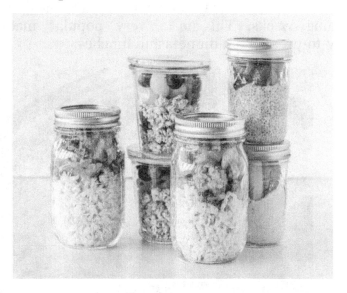

- **Ready prepared ingredients:** This form of meal prep is perfect for those of us who still enjoy cooking our meals but may be short on time or energy to prepare ingredients. With this form of meal prep, we'll ready all the ingredients we need for meals long beforehand and refrigerate them.

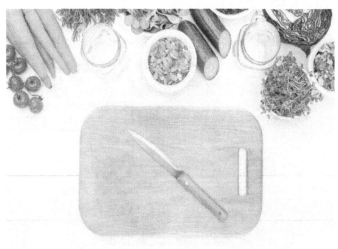

The method that is best for you really depends on how much time you have and what your daily routine is. For example, your commute to work may be very short, so breakfast is never eaten in a rush. But, because of your long work hours, you'd like to prepare your dinners ahead of time.

In this case, we could prepare make-ahead meals for your dinner to help streamline your day and allow you time to relax when you get home from a busy day. Another example could be you have very little time in the mornings to worry about breakfast and lunch for yourself, so you could prepare some individual meal portions ahead of time to keep you going throughout the day.

- Food Storage Tips:

  - When storing food in general, make sure your refrigerator temperature is at least 40°F or lower and your freezer should be at least 0°F or lower.
  - After cooking meals, it is best to allow them to cool down to room temperature before putting them in the refrigerator or freezer.
  - Glass containers are incredibly useful for storing meals because you can see what is inside without having to open them and break the airtight seal.

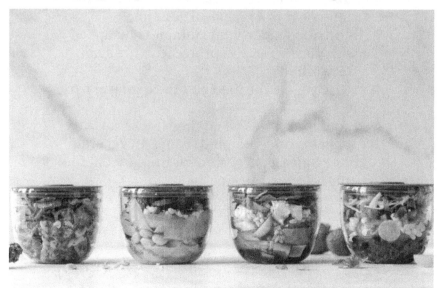

- If you use plastic containers, make sure they are BPA free and microwave safe.
- When defrosting meals, leaving it in the fridge overnight is the safest and most effective way. Otherwise, placing the frozen container into room temperature water will also speed up the defrosting process. Microwaving should be a last resort as it may overcook the food in some areas and leave an unsatisfying result.

- Fridge or Freezer:

First, Check the expiration of your ingredients as you go. If you use yogurt about to expire tomorrow in a recipe today, then that recipe that is always good for 3 days, may be bad tomorrow.

Once food has been cooked, it's generally considered edible for 3 to 5 days. If you think you won't use it in that time, throw it in the freezer to eat later. However, I regularly meal prep for up to extend the shelf life of your meal-prepped foods.

A few tips for freezer success are:

- Freeze meals in individual portions so you can reheat just one meal at a time.
- Store food in airtight containers, wrapped with plastic wrap to protect further against freezer burn.
- Clearly label the food and the date you froze it.
- Liquids expands when they freeze, so leave room in the container for this. In general, leave at least 40 percent of the container empty for expansion.

	FRIDGE	FREEZER
Raw poultry	1 to 2 days	9 months
Fresh, raw fish	1 to 2 days	2 to 3 months
Uncooked tofu	7 days	5 months
Soups and stews	3 to 4 days	2 to 3 months
Cooked dishes with eggs, poultry, or fish	3 to 4 days	2 to 3 months
Cooked beans	6 to 7 days	6 to 12 months
Cooked grains	4 to 6 days	6 months
Salads: egg, chicken, fish	3 to 4 days	Not recommended
Hard-cooked eggs	7 days	Not recommended

Chapter 3: Shopping List

Week One

This list outlines everything you need to make all the recipes for the week, plus all the sides and snacks for ONE person to follow the plan.

Shopping List — Week ONE

Shop for:

Vegetables
- 2 cups crimini mushrooms
- 8 loosely packed baby spinach leaves, chopped
- 1/2 cup tomatoes with 8 cherry tomatoes
- 1 cucumber
- 2 cups of carrot
- 1 small zucchini

Bread:
- 4 large whole wheat tortillas
- Whole-wheat bread, toasted

Dairy:
- 1/4 cup + 2 tablespoons cheese
- Low-fat mozzarella cheese
- 4 ounce fat-free cottage cheese
- 1/3 cup freshly grated Parmigiano-Reggiano cheese

Meat& Seafoods:
- 13 ounces salmon
- 3 chicken breasts
- 1/2 canned chicken
- Low sodium chicken broth

Herbs:
- Cilantro
- Parsley
- Oregano

Check Your Pantry For:

Oils, Vinegars & Condiments:
- Canola oil
- Olive oil, extra-virgin
- Honey
- Soy Sauce
- Hoisin sauce
- Sesame oil
- Cooking Spray, non-stick

Flavouring
- Salt
- Low-fat monterey Jack cheese
- Onions, white, red & green
- Sriracha
- Sugar
- Garlic
- Cinnamon
- Ground cumin
- 1 teaspoon vanilla extract
- Fat free mayonnaise
- Ground pepper, black
- Basil, dried
- Fresh chives
- Jalapeno chile peppers

Dry Goods:
- Old-fashioned rolled oats
- 2/3 cup packed Medjool dates
- 2 teaspoons cornstarch
- 1/8 teaspoon garlic powder
- 2 teaspoons curry powder
- Paprika

Nuts, Seeds & Fruits:
- 1/2 medium-size ripe banana
- 1 teaspoon chia seeds
- 1/4 cup frozen thawed mixed berries
- 1 tablespoon chopped walnuts
- 1/2 cup dried blueberries
- 1/2 cup of quinoa
- Apple
- 1 cup corn kernel
- 70g green beans
- 2 ripe avocado
- Poppy seeds
- Pecans
- 1/2 cup squah, yellow
- Lemon
- Raisin, golden
- 2 almonds

Refrigerator Items:
- 2 cups plain 2% reduced-fat Greek yogurt
- 2/3 cup unsweetened almond milk
- 1 tablespoon cider vinegar
- Eggs
- Low-fat milk
- Frozen stir-fry vegetables
- Fresh lemon juice
- Butter milk

Week Two

This list outlines everything you need to make all the recipes for the week, plus all the sides and snacks for ONE person to follow the plan.

Shopping List Week Two

Shop for:

Vegetables:
- 2 cups package microwaveable Broccoli florets
- Cauliflower florets
- 2 cups scallions
- 2 cups broccoli with stems
- Cherry tomatoes
- Zucchini
- 1/2 red cabbage
- Carrots
- Cucumber
- 1/4 cup spinach
- Lettuce, romaine

Herbs:
- Fresh tarragon
- Arugula
- Grounded ginger
- Fresh mint
- Parsley
- Oregano
- Cilantro
- Chivas

Bread & Rolls:
- Crusty whole wheat bread
- 2 tortillas
- Rice papers
- 8 eaches 6-inch flour tortillas
- 1 (9-inch) Whole wheat pie-crust shell

Dairy:
- Sharp cheddar cheese
- Cottage cheese
- 1/4 cup part skim shredded mozzarella cheese
- Reduced-fat swiss cheese

Meat:
- Chicken in breast
- Boneless skinless chicken thighs
- Shredded chicken
- 1 pound pork loin
- 2 boneless pork chops

Check Your Pantry For:

Oils, Vinegars & Condiments:
- Olive oil
- Sesame oil
- Olive oil spray
- Red wine vinegar
- Rice vinegar
- White vinegar
- Hoisin sauce
- 1/2 teaspoon apple cider
- Mustard powder, dijon
- Soy sauce, gluten-free
- Fish sauce
- Light mayonnaise
- Extra-virgin olive oil
- Honey

Flavouring:
- Kosher salt
- Sugar
- Curry powder
- Shallots
- Ground cardamon
- Thyme
- Ground pepper, black and red
- Cumin
- Fresh basil, julienned
- Monterey Jack cheese
- vanilla extract
- Brown sugar
- Grounded cinnamon
- Onion, red
- Sriracha
- Sea salt

Nuts, Seeds & Fruits:
- 1/2 cup cream & smooth peanut butter
- 1/4 cup ground flax seeds
- 5 Lemon
- Capsicum
- 1 jar pimento
- Quinoa
- 1 cup walnuts
- Dried cranberries
- 1 Apple
- Seedless grapes
- Raisins
- Chocolate granola
- 1/4 avocado
- Chia seeds

Dry Goods:
- Old fashioned Oats
- 1 cup brown rice
- Garlic powder
- Onion powder
- Thai chilies
- Chili powder
- 1/4 semi-sweet chocolate chips

Refrigerator Items:
- Eggs
- Evapored milk
- Reduced-fat sour cream
- Lemon juice
- Raspberry yogurt
- 1/8 cup fresh low-fat curds
- 1/2 cup whole milk
- Reduced-fat milk

Week Three

This list outlines everything you need to make all the recipes for the week, plus all the sides and snacks for ONE person to follow the plan.

Shopping List Week Three

Shop for:

Vegetables:
- Fresh & canned tomatoes
- Small cauliflower florets
- 1/2 cup broccoli florets
- 1 teaspoon chopped fresh sage
- 5 ounces potato gnocchi
- 1/2 cup shredded cabbage
- 5 ounces romaine leaves
- Fresh cremini mushrooms
- 3 stalks celery
- 1/4 cup hummus
- Baby spinach leaves
- Okra
- Cucumber
- 3 carrots

Bread & Wheat Flour:
- 1 1/2 whole wheat pita bread
- 3 cups bread flour
- 1 whole wheat frankfurter buns
- 3 ounces whole-wheat spaghetti

Herbs:
- Dried rosemary
- Parsley, Italian
- Oregano

Meat & Seafoods:
- 1 Boneless skinless chicken breast
- 1/2 low-sodium & 32 ounces chicken broth
- 1/2 pound boneless skinless chicken thighs
- 2 ounces turkey meatballs
- 1/2 pound ground turkey
- 6 ounces salmon filet

Dairy:
- Feta cheese
- Parmesan cheese
- Reduced-fat mozzarella cheese

Oils, Vinegars & Condiments:
- Maple syrup
- Dijon mustard
- Honey
- White wine vinegar
- Olive oil
- 1 cup butter
- Extra-virgin olive oil
- Balsamic vinegar

Flavouring:
- Fresh basil
- Kosher salt
- Ground cinnamon
- Ground turmeric
- Ground pepper, red, green & black
- Half & half
- Fresh red bell pepper
- Saffron
- Vanilla extract
- Italian seasoning
- Salt

Dry Goods:
- Old-fashioned rolled oats
- All-purpose flour
- 2/3 cup packed Medjool dates
- 3 teaspoons active dry yeast
- Garlic powder
- Parmesan flakes
- Paprika

Check Your Pantry For:

Nuts, Seeds & Fruits:
- Avocado
- Kalamata olives
- Butternut spaush
- Ground flaxseeds
- 1 lime
- Chia seeds
- Brown rice (jasmine or basmati)
- 1/2 cup lentils
- Granola oats
- 1 can fresh cannellini beans
- Blueberries
- 1 medium banana
- Pecans
- Apple
- Whole almonds

Refrigerator Items:
- Eggs
- 1 cup Greek yogurt
- Skim milk
- Refrigerated pesto
- Unsweetened almond milk
- Tomato sauce
- Nonfat, artificially sweetened vanilla yogurt
- 1 cup ice cubes
- Fresh lemon juice

38

Week Four

This list outlines everything you need to make all the recipes for the week, plus all the sides and snacks for ONE person to follow the plan.

Shopping List Week Four

Shop for:

Vegetables:
- Baby spinach
- 1 package mixed vegetables
- 1 pound beef
- 1/2 pound broccoli
- 2 radishes
- Cucumber
- Tomatoes
- 1/2 medium zucchini
- Romaine lettuce
- Sweet potatoes
- 1/4 pound baby red-skinned potatoes
- 1/2 cup chopped cabbage

Herbs:
- Fresh parsley
- Fennel
- Fresh rosemary
- Cilantro

Bread & Wheat Flour:
- 3 6-inch whole-wheat or corn tortillas
- Pita, for serving

Dairy:
- Grated parmesan cheese
- Monterey Jack Cheese
- 1/4 low-fat cottage cheese

Meat & Seafoods:
- 12 ounces beef tenderloin or filet mignon
- 1 steak
- 2 ounces of smoked salmon
- 1 6-ounces filets tilapia, cod, barramundi, or other flaky white fish
- 1/2 pound orange roughy fish fillets
- 2 skin-on trout filets

Check Your Pantry For:

Oils, Vinegars & Condiments:
- Cooking Spray, non-stick
- Olive oil
- Unsalted butter
- Extra olive oil
- Honey
- Spicy maple syrup
- Sherry vinegar
- Canola oil

Flavouring
- Salt
- Sea salt
- Onion, red & green
- Bell pepper
- Kosher salt
- Salsa
- Sugar
- Thyme
- Taco seasoning
- Olives
- Ground coriander
- Ground cumin
- Ground cinnamon
- Pepper, black & red
- Vanilla extract

Dry Goods:
- 1/3 cup rolled oats
- White whole wheat flour
- Baking powder
- Chili powder
- Baking soda
- Garlic powder

Nuts, Seeds & Fruits:
- Blueberries
- Canned garbanzo beans with canned black beans
- Fresh avocado
- White rice
- Green chilies
- Tahini
- Lemon zest
- Apples
- 1/2 cup chopped walnuts
- 1/2 banana
- 1 tablespoon chia seeds

Refrigerator Items:
- Eggs
- Egg whites
- Buttermilk
- Queso Fresco
- Plain nonfat Greek yogurt
- 1/3 cup milk
- Lemon juice

Chapter 4: Diabetic Meal Plan for Four Weeks?

When preparing a week" worth of meals, the most important thing to consider is variety. We don't want to get bored with our food, and we want to make sure we are getting a balanced variety of nutrients. When prepping your meals for a week, try to cook a few different types of recipes.

A good seven-day plan will include breakfast, lunch, and dinner for all the days of the week, as well as healthy snacks. Keep in mind, you should always take into account your calorific needs. Not everybody has the same needs when it comes to calorie intake, and depending on your age, gender, level of activity, and whether you want to lose weight, you may need less or more than the recommended amount.

Something important to note as a diabetic is the right time to eat. Consistently eating at the same time every day is key to keeping a steady blood sugar level. As well as eating at the same time, it is recommended that you don't go more than four hours without eating.

I included numbers after each day; you'll find out why they are there in the week's prep section.

Week One

Monday (1) Week One	Daily Total: Calories: 1197 Kcal Carbs: 78.2g Sugar: 23.3g
Breakfast:	Overnight oatmeal with berries and nuts
Morning Snack:	Half a cup of mixed nuts and berries
Lunch:	Spinach rolls
Afternoon Snack:	No-bake blueberry oat bites
Dinner:	Salmon and spinach with avocado

Overnight oatmeal with berries and nuts **(Pg. 58)**
Spinach rolls **(Pg. 103)**
Salmon and spinach with avocado **(Pg. 155)**

Tuesday (2) Week One	Daily Total: Calories: 698.5 Kcal Carbs: 48 g Sugar: 12.8 g
Breakfast:	Mushroom breakfast burrito
Morning Snack:	A sliced apple with cinnamon
Lunch:	Smoked salmon wrap
Afternoon Snack:	Spinach rolls
Dinner:	Spicy chicken and quinoa

Mushroom breakfast burrito **(Pg. 60)**
Smoked salmon wrap **(Pg. 106)**
Spicy chicken and quinoa **(Pg. 161)**

Wednesday(3) Week One	Daily Total: Calories: 1084 Kcal Carbs: 108.4 g Sugar: 23.7 g
Breakfast:	No-bake blueberry oat bites
Morning Snack:	Half a cup of Greek yogurt with fresh blueberries
Lunch:	Spinach rolls
Afternoon Snack:	No-bake protein bar
Dinner:	Salmon with quinoa and vegetable stir fry

No-bake blueberry oat bites **(Pg. 62)**
Spinach rolls **(Pg. 103)**
Salmon with quinoa and vegetable stir fry **(Pg. 157)**

Thursday(4) Week One	Daily Total: Calories: 655 Kcal Carbs: 49 g Sugar: 8 g
Breakfast:	Mushroom breakfast burrito
Morning Snack:	A small bunch of grapes
Lunch:	Smoked salmon wrap
Afternoon Snack:	Celery with nut butter
Dinner:	Chicken and vegetable stir fry

Mushroom breakfast burrito **(Pg. 60)**
Smoked salmon wrap **(Pg. 106)**
Chicken and vegetable stir fry **(Pg. 159)**

Friday(5) Week One	Daily Total: Calories: 669 Kcal Carbs: 39.7 g Sugar: 10.5 g
Breakfast:	Avocado and egg on whole wheat toast
Morning Snack:	A banana with nut butter
Lunch:	Chicken and egg salad bowl
Afternoon Snack:	No-bake blueberry oat bites
Dinner:	Spicy chicken and quinoa

Avocado and egg on whole wheat toast **(Pg. 64)**
Chicken and egg salad bowl **(Pg. 108)**
Spicy chicken and quinoa **(Pg. 161)**

Saturday(6) Week One	Daily Total: Calories: 895.5 Kcal Carbs: 63.9 g Sugar: 37.2 g
Breakfast:	A cup of cottage cheese with peach slices
Morning Snack:	Peach slices and half a cup of mixed nuts
Lunch:	Leftover spicy chicken sandwich
Afternoon Snack:	No-bake protein bar
Dinner:	Spinach, apple, and chicken salad

A cup of cottage cheese with peach slices **(Pg. 66)**
Leftover spicy chicken sandwich **(Pg. 110)**
Spinach, apple, and chicken salad **(Pg. 163)**

Sunday(7) Week One	Daily Total: Calories: 844.2 Kcal Carbs: 3.9 g Sugar: 77.2 g
Breakfast:	Stir-fried vegetable and egg omelet
Morning Snack:	A boiled egg and cottage cheese
Lunch:	Greek yogurt with apple and cinnamon
Afternoon Snack:	A tangerine, orange, or other type of citrus fruit
Dinner:	Leafy green salmon salad with sesame seeds

Stir-fried vegetable and egg omelet **(Pg. 72)**
Greek yogurt with apple and cinnamon **(Pg. 112)**
Leafy green salmon salad with sesame seeds **(Pg. 165)**

Prep for Week One

Meal preparations for week one are very simple. The numbers in brackets correlate to the days in which the prepared food will be consumed. A breakdown of our prep is as follows:

- Batch cooking chicken (2, 4, 5, 6) and quinoa (2, 3, 5) separately
- Prepare two mushroom breakfast burritos (2, 4) for refrigeration
- Prepare and refrigerating no-bake blueberry oat bites (1, 3, 5) and no-bake protein bars (3, 6)
- Bake spinach rolls (1, 2, 3) for at least three days of lunch and snacks
- Prepare a large, multi-portion leafy green salad bowl (5, 6, 7)
- Portion and package smoked salmon (1, 2, 3, 4 , 7)
- Prepare salmon wraps for at least two days of lunch (2, 4)
- Stir fry mixed vegetables (3, 4, 7)

Week Two

Monday (1) Week Two	Daily Total: Calories: 800.5 Kcal Carbs: 30 g Sugar: 10.7 g
Breakfast:	Made-ahead breakfast quiche
Morning Snack:	A tangerine, orange, or other type of citrus fruit
Lunch:	Chicken salad bowl with olive oil dressing
Afternoon Snack:	A sliced apple with cinnamon
Dinner:	Rosemary pork chops with roasted cauliflower

Made-ahead breakfast quiche **(Pg. 76)**
Chicken salad bowl with olive oil dressing **(Pg. 114)**
Rosemary pork chops with roasted cauliflower **(Pg. 168)**

Tuesday (2) Week Two	Daily Total: Calories: 999 Kcal Carbs: 90.5 g Sugar: 17.7 g
Breakfast:	No-bake nut butter protein bites
Morning Snack:	Peach slices and half a cup of mixed nuts
Lunch:	Spicy pork on a whole wheat roll
Afternoon Snack:	Half a cup of Greek yogurt with fresh blueberries
Dinner:	Grilled chicken with roasted cauliflower and quinoa

No-bake nut butter protein bites **(Pg. 84)**
Spicy pork on a whole wheat roll **(Pg. 116)**
Grilled chicken with roasted cauliflower and quinoa **(Pg. 170)**

Wednesday (3) Week Two	Daily Total: Calories: 617 Kcal Carbs: 41.4 g Sugar: 8.2 g
Breakfast:	Made-ahead breakfast quiche
Morning Snack:	No-bake nut butter protein bites
Lunch:	Green salad with creamy dressing
Afternoon Snack:	A banana with nut butter
Dinner:	Grilled chicken chopped salad

Made-ahead breakfast quiche **(Pg. 76)**
Green salad with creamy dressing **(Pg. 119)**
Grilled chicken chopped salad **(Pg. 173)**

Thursday (4) Week Two	Daily Total: Calories: 563.9 Kcal Carbs: 41.4 g Sugar: 9.9 g
Breakfast:	Chicken on whole wheat toast with olive oil
Morning Snack:	A tangerine, orange, or other type of citrus fruit
Lunch:	A cup of Greek yogurt with berries and chia seeds
Afternoon Snack:	No-bake nut butter protein bites
Dinner:	Thai stir fry with pork strips

Chicken on whole wheat toast with olive oil **(Pg. 86)**
A cup of Greek yogurt with berries and chia seeds **(Pg. 121)**
Thai stir fry with pork strips **(Pg. 176)**

Friday (5) Week Two	Daily Total: Calories: 334 Kcal Carbs: 28 g Sugar: 8 g
Breakfast:	No-bake nut butter protein bites
Morning Snack:	A bunch of grapes
Lunch:	A cup of cottage cheese with olive oil and diced cherry tomatoes
Afternoon Snack:	A small cup of muesli and Greek yogurt
Dinner:	Spicy pork tacos

No-bake nut butter protein bites **(Pg. 84)**
A cup of cottage cheese with olive oil and diced cherry tomatoes **(Pg. 123)**
Spicy pork tacos **(Pg. 178)**

Saturday (6) Week Two	Daily Total: Calories: 917.3 Kcal Carbs: 83.8 g Sugar: 21.5 g
Breakfast:	Avocado and egg on whole wheat toast
Morning Snack:	A diced pear
Lunch:	Chicken and salad wrap
Afternoon Snack:	Celery with nut butter
Dinner:	Chicken and quinoa one pot with broccoli

Avocado and egg on whole wheat toast **(Pg. 64)**
Chicken and salad wrap **(Pg. 125)**
Chicken and quinoa one pot with broccoli **(Pg. 180)**

Sunday (7) Week Two	Daily Total: Calories: 816.7 Kcal Carbs: 56.2 g Sugar: 28.6 g
Breakfast:	Broccoli omelet
Morning Snack:	Half a cup of mixed nuts and berries
Lunch:	Apple and cottage cheese salad
Afternoon Snack:	An assortment of cheese and crackers
Dinner:	Chicken and vegetable bowl with cottage cheese

Broccoli omelet **(Pg. 88)**
Apple and cottage cheese salad **(Pg. 127)**
Chicken and vegetable bowl with cottage cheese **(Pg. 182)**

Prep for Week Two

Week two's meal preparations focus on a lot of made-ahead meals; a breakdown of our prep is as follows:

- Batch cooking chicken (1, 2, 3, 4, 6, 7), pork (1, 2, 4, 5) cauliflower (1, 2), and broccoli (6, 7)
- Bake the breakfast quiche (1, 3)
- Prepare the no-bake nut butter protein bites (2, 3, 4, 5)
- Prepare a large, multi-portion leafy green salad bowl (1, 3, 6, 7)
- Cook and portion the quinoa (2, 6)

Monday (1) Week Three	Daily Total: Calories: 1533.5 Kcal Carbs: 63.1 g Sugar: 22.7g
Breakfast:	Egg and avocado omelet
Morning Snack:	Half a cup of mixed nuts and berries
Lunch:	Hummus and green salad
Afternoon Snack:	Celery and nut butter
Dinner:	Slow cooker vegetable soup with whole wheat toast

Egg and avocado omelet (Pg. 90)
Hummus and green salad (Pg. 129)
Slow cooker vegetable soup with whole wheat toast (Pg. 133)

Tuesday (2) Week Three	Daily Total: Calories: 717.3 Kcal Carbs: 85.8 g Sugar: 17.8 g
Breakfast:	Apple and cinnamon overnight oats
Morning Snack:	A diced pear
Lunch:	Chicken and cauliflower salad bowl
Afternoon Snack:	Ham and cheese on whole wheat crackers
Dinner:	Lentils and green salad with dressing

Apple and cinnamon overnight oats (Pg. 92)
Chicken and cauliflower salad bowl (Pg. 131)
Lentils and green salad with dressing (Pg. 184)

Wednesday (3) Week Three	Daily Total: Calories: 1078.3 Kcal Carbs: 84.4 g Sugar: 13.9 g
Breakfast:	Apple and cinnamon overnight oats
Morning Snack:	A tangerine, orange, or other type of citrus fruit
Lunch:	Chicken and cauliflower salad bowl
Afternoon Snack:	Half a cup of Greek yogurt with an apple
Dinner:	Salmon and pepper with green salad

Apple and cinnamon overnight oats (Pg. 92)
Chicken and cauliflower salad bowl (Pg. 131)
Salmon and pepper with green salad (Pg. 186)

Thursday (4) Week Three	Daily Total: Calories: 1142.7 Kcal Carbs: 44.4 g Sugar: 28.7 g
Breakfast:	No-bake blueberry oat bites
Morning Snack:	A boiled egg with cottage
Lunch:	Slow cooker vegetable soup with whole wheat toast
Afternoon Snack:	A banana with nut butter
Dinner:	Lemon and herb chicken with brown rice

No-bake blueberry oat bites (Pg. 62)
Slow cooker vegetable soup with whole wheat toast (Pg. 129)
Lemon and herb chicken with brown rice (Pg. 188)

Friday (5) Week Three	Daily Total: Calories: 1239.8 Kcal Carbs: 67.3 g Sugar: 24.3 g
Breakfast:	Apple and cinnamon overnight oats
Morning Snack:	No-bake blueberry oat bites
Lunch:	Slow cooker vegetable soup with whole wheat toast
Afternoon Snack:	Peach slices and half a cup of mixed nuts
Dinner:	Whole wheat spaghetti and meatballs

Apple and cinnamon overnight oats **(Pg. 92)**
Slow cooker vegetable soup with whole wheat toast **(Pg. 129)**
Whole wheat spaghetti and meatballs **(Pg. 191)**

Saturday (6) Week Three	Daily Total: Calories: 912 Kcal Carbs: 97 g Sugar: 17 g
Breakfast:	No-bake blueberry oat bites
Morning Snack:	Half a cup of no-added sugar muesli and Greek yogurt
Lunch:	Meatballs in a whole wheat bun
Afternoon Snack:	Half a cup of mixed nuts
Dinner:	Grilled chicken with spinach and butternut

No-bake blueberry oats bites **(Pg. 62)**
Meatballs in a whole wheat bun **(Pg. 136)**
Grilled chicken with spinach and butternut **(Pg. 193)**

Sunday (7) Week Three	Daily Total: Calories: 744.5 Kcal Carbs: 96.5 g Sugar: 0 g
Breakfast:	Banana and berry smoothie
Morning Snack:	A tangerine, orange, or other type of citrus fruit
Lunch:	A bowl of Greek yogurt with mixed nuts and berries
Afternoon Snack:	No-bakes blueberry oat bites
Dinner:	Whole wheat spaghetti and meatballs

Banana and berry smoothie **(Pg. 74)**
A bowl of Greek yogurt with mixed nuts and berries **(Pg. 138)**
Whole wheat spaghetti and meatballs **(Pg. 191)**

Prep for Week Three

Week three's meal preparations are as follows:

- Slow cook the vegetable soup (1, 4, 5)
- Batch cook whole wheat spaghetti and meatballs (5, 6, 7) and chicken (2, 3, 4, 6)
- Prepare and refrigerate the no-bake blueberry oat bites (4, 5, 6, 7)
- Prepare and refrigerate the apple and cinnamon overnight oats (2, 3, 5)
- Prepare the chicken and cauliflower salad bowls (2, 3)
- Prepare a large, multi-portion leafy green salad bowl (1, 2, 3)

Monday (1) Week Four	Daily Total: Calories: 780 Kcal Carbs: 64.6 g Sugar: 5.2 g
Breakfast:	Egg muffins
Morning Snack:	Half a cup of mixed nuts and berries
Lunch:	Bean and beef taco bowl
Afternoon Snack:	No-bakes protein bar
Dinner:	Pan seared trout with stir fried vegetables

Egg Muffins (Pg. 94)
Bean and beef taco bowl (Pg. 140)
Pan seared trout with stir fried vegetables (Pg. 195)

Tuesday (2) Week Four	Daily Total: Calories: 1006 Kcal Carbs: 92.4 g Sugar: 1.2 g
Breakfast:	Blueberry and nut overnight oats
Morning Snack:	A cup of cottage cheese and cherry tomatoes
Lunch:	Pepper and cottage cheese salad bowl
Afternoon Snack:	Half a cup of baby carrots
Dinner:	Beef strips and stir-fried vegetables

Blueberry and nut overnight oats (Pg. 96)
Pepper and cottage cheese salad bowl (Pg. 142)
Beef strips and stir-fried vegetables (Pg. 197)

Wednesday (3) Week Four	Daily Total: Calories: 905 Kcal Carbs: 84 g Sugar: 9 g
Breakfast:	Egg muffins
Morning Snack:	No-bake protein bar
Lunch:	Bean and beef taco bowl
Afternoon Snack:	A diced apple with cinnamon
Dinner:	Fish tacos with salad

Egg Muffins (Pg. 94)
Bean and beef taco bowl (Pg. 140)
Fish tacos with salad (Pg. 206)

Thursday (4) Week Four	Daily Total: Calories: 1031 Kcal Carbs: 108.42 g Sugar: 1.2 g
Breakfast:	Blueberry and nut overnight oats
Morning Snack:	A hard-boiled egg with chili oil
Lunch:	Pepper and cottage cheese salad bowl
Afternoon Snack:	A tangerine, orange, or other type of citrus fruit
Dinner:	Steak and sautéed zucchini

Blueberry and nut overnight oats (Pg. 96)
Pepper and cottage cheese salad bowl (Pg. 142)
Steak and sauteed zucchini (Pg. 201)

Friday (5) Week Four	Daily Total: Calories: 1734 Kcal Carbs: 172 g Sugar: 19 g
Breakfast:	Blueberry and nut overnight oats
Morning Snack:	Half a cup of Greek yogurt and dried berries
Lunch:	Bean and beef taco bowl
Afternoon Snack:	No-bake protein bar
Dinner:	Steak with sweet potato and broccoli

Blueberry and nut overnight oats **(Pg. 96)**
Bean and beef taco bowl **(Pg. 140)**
Steak with sweet potato and broccoli **(Pg. 203)**

Saturday (6) Week Four	Daily Total: Calories: 854.99 Kcal Carbs: 61.38 g Sugar: 5.33 g
Breakfast:	Egg muffins
Morning Snack:	No-bake protein bar
Lunch:	Pepper and cottage cheese salad bowl
Afternoon Snack:	Half a cup of Greek yogurt and a diced peach
Dinner:	Fish tacos with stir-fried vegetables

Egg Muffins **(Pg. 94)**
Pepper and cottage cheese salad bowl **(Pg. 142)**
Fish tacos with stir-fried vegetables **(Pg. 206)**

Sunday (7) Week Four	Daily Total: Calories: 592 Kcal Carbs: 57.74 g Sugar: 7.55 g
Breakfast:	Apple and cinnamon pancakes
Morning Snack:	Half a cup of mixed nuts and berries
Lunch:	Avocado and egg on whole wheat toast with chili oil
Afternoon Snack:	A banana with nut butter
Dinner:	Hummus and olive oil salad with cottage cheese

Apple and cinnamon pancakes **(Pg. 98)**
Avocado and egg on whole wheat toast with chili oil **(Pg. 144)**
Hummus and olive oil salad with cottage cheese **(Pg. 208)**

Prep for Week Four

Week four's meal prep is as follows:

- Batch cook the trout (1, 3, 6) and beef (1, 2, 3, 4, 5)
- Prepare and refrigerate the no-bake protein bars (1, 3, 5, 6)
- Bake the egg muffins (1, 3, 6)
- Prepare the bean and beef taco bowls (1, 3, 5)
- Prepare the pepper and cottage cheese salad bowls (2, 4, 6)
- Prepare and refrigerate the blueberry and nut overnight oats (2, 4, 5)

Chapter 5: Recipes for Diabetic

Cooking Measurement Chart

Weight		Measurement				Temperature	
imperial	metric	cup	onces	milliliters	tbsp.	fahrenheit	celsius
1/2 oz	15 g	8 cup	64 oz	1895 ml	128	100 °F	37 °C
1 oz	29 g	6 cup	48 oz	1420 ml	96	150 °F	65 °C
2 oz	57 g	5 cup	40 oz	1180 ml	80	200 °F	93 °C
3 oz	85 g	4 cup	32 oz	960 ml	64	250 °F	121 °C
4 oz	113 g	2 cup	16 oz	480 ml	32	300 °F	150 °C
5 oz	141 g	1 cup	8 oz	240 ml	16	325 °F	160 °C
6 oz	170 g	3/4 cup	6 oz	177 ml	12	350 °F	180 °C
8 oz	227 g	2/3 cup	5 oz	158 ml	11	375 °F	190 °C
10 oz	283 g	1/2 cup	4 oz	118 ml	8	400 °F	200 °C
12 oz	340 g	3/8 cup	3 oz	90 ml	6	425 °F	220 °C
13 oz	369 g	1/3 cup	2.5 oz	79 ml	5.5	450 °F	230 °C
14 oz	397 g	1/4 cup	2 oz	59 ml	4	500 °F	260 °C
15 oz	425 g	1/8 cup	1 oz	30 ml	3	525 °F	274 °C
1 lb	453 g	1/16 cup	1/2 oz	15 ml	1	550 °F	288 °C

Breakfast Recipes

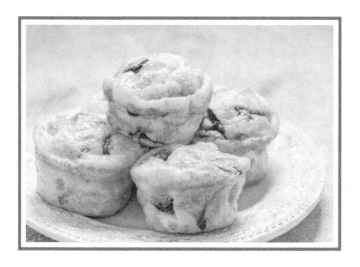

Overnight Oatmeal With Berries And Nuts

Cook Time:
0 minutes

Prep Time:
5 minutes

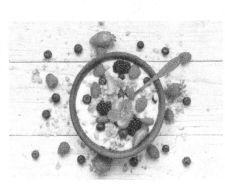

Serving Size
1
**Calories
per serving:**
359kcal
**Carbs
per serving:**
52g

Speed up your morning routine with this nutritious breakfast recipe made the night before. This is a naturally sweetened recipe packed with fruits and a pro-biotic boost from the Greek Yogurt, which will keep your mornings low-maintenance without skimping on flavor or fuel.

Per Serving:

Fat: 13g | **Saturated fat:** 2g
Protein: 14g | **Fiber:** 10g |
Sodium: 397mg | **Calcium:** 26%
DV | **Potassium:** 16% DV | **Sugar:** 14g

Tip:

Refrigerate the mixture overnight, and top with berries and walnuts.

Ingredients:

- 1/2 medium-size ripe banana
- 1/8 teaspoon of kosher salt
- 2/3 cup of unsweetened almond milk
- 1/4 cup of frozen-thawed mixed berries
- 1 tablespoon of chopped walnuts
- 1/4 cup of plain 2% reduced-fat Greek yogurt
- 1/2 cup of old-fashioned rolled oats
- 1 teaspoon of chia seeds

Direction:

1. In a small bowl, place the banana, and use a fork to mash it thoroughly.
2. Add yogurt and mix to combine.
3. Add chia seeds, oats, salt, and almond milk.
4. Mix well and cover.
5. Refrigerate over the night or at least 6 hours.
6. Top with mixed berries and walnuts.
7. Serve and enjoy.

Mushroom Breakfast Burrito

Cook Time:
20 minutes

Prep Time:
10 minutes

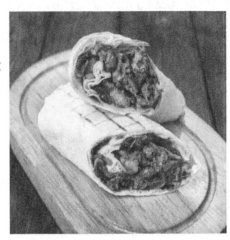

Serving Size
1
Calories per serving:
385kcal
Carbs per serving:
28g

Having Mushroom in your morning diet is so great. Mushrooms have a savory umami flavor that amps up the taste of any dish. You need to whip up a batch of these healthy vegetarian Mushroom Breakfast Burrito today, so you can have an energizing and healthy breakfast at your fingertips in minutes. Enjoy!

Per Serving:

Fat: 22g | Saturated fat: 6g
Protein: 20g | Fiber: 4g |
Sodium: 640mg | Calcium: 21%
DV | Potassium: 487mg | Sugar:
4g

Tip:

After freezing, place on a microwave-safe dish and microwave until heated through, for about 2 minutes.

Ingredients:

- 0.5 tablespoons of neutral oil canola, vegetable, grape-seed
- 0.13 white onion diced
- 0.5 garlic clove minced
- 0.5 cups of crimini mushrooms chopped
- Cooking spray
- 1 large whole wheat tortillas
- 0.06 cup + 2 tablespoons of goat cheese
- 1 cups of loosely packed spinach chopped
- 0.06 teaspoon of salt
- 2 large eggs
- 0.75 tablespoons of milk
- Salt and pepper to taste

Direction:

1. Add oil to the pan in a large skillet over medium-high heat.
2. Add the garlic, onion and cook until translucent, for about 2 to 3 minutes. Add the mushrooms, then cook for 3 minutes, until they are golden brown.
3. Flip the mushrooms to allow the other side to cook.
4. In the pan, place spinach and cook for about 3 to 4 minutes, until it's wilted. Season with salt and stir all the veggies together. Remove from the heat, then set it aside.
5. Whisk together milk and eggs in a large bowl. Season with pepper and salt to taste.
6. Over medium heat, heat another large skillet, spray the skillet using cooking spray. Add egg mixture, then cook until the eggs have set, frequently stirring, for about 4 to 5 minutes. Remove from heat.
7. In the microwave, heat the tortillas for 10 seconds.
8. On a piece of aluminum foil, layout the tortillas and spread half tablespoon of goat cheese on it.
9. Distribute the roasted vegetables and scrambled eggs evenly.
10. Roll up in the foil, and place it in a freezer bag. Then freeze.
11. Unwrap the burritos from the foil when ready to eat from the freezer. Serve and enjoy.

No-Bake Blueberry Oat Bites

Cook Time:
0 minutes

Prep Time:
10 minutes

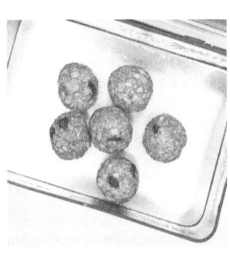

Serving Size
1
Calories per serving:
101kcal
Carbs per serving:
15g

No-Bake Blueberry Oats Bites are 7-ingredients healthy snacks that are easy and super addictive. The most exciting part of these bites are they are diabetic friendly, vegan, and gluten-free.
You can easily double this recipe if you're making these for a bigger group.
It's certain they would love it!

Per Serving:

Fat: 0g | **Saturated fat:** 0g
Protein: 0g | **Fiber:** 1g | **Sodium:** 14mg | **Calcium:** 0% DV | **Potassium:** 0% DV | **Sugar:** 13g

Tip:

Store extra cookie balls in the refrigerator in an airtight container for up to 7 days.

Ingredients:

- 1 cup of old-fashioned rolled
- 2/3 cup of packed Medjool dates, pitted and chopped (about 7-8 large ones)
- 1 teaspoon of vanilla extract
- pinch of salt
- 1-3 tablespoons of water, as needed
- 1/2 cup of dried blueberries
- 1 teaspoon of fresh lemon juice

Direction:

1) In your food processor, add all of the ingredients together.
2) Wait and scrape down the sides as needed. Do this until it's well-combined.
3) Add more water if you want to get the mixture to come together.
4) Wet hands.
5) Roll mixture into golf ball-sized cookie balls.
6) Serve immediately or cover and refrigerate.
7) Enjoy!

Avocado And Egg On Whole Wheat Toast

Cook Time:
0 minutes

Prep Time:
5 minutes

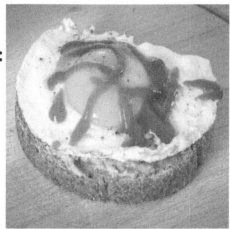

Serving Size
1
Calories per serving:
270.9kcal
Carbs per serving:
18.1g

If you can try this recipe once, you will agree that topping avocado toast with an egg is a near-perfect breakfast. This recipe is very filling, and you'll want to add it to your favorite breakfast.

Per Serving:

Fat: 17.7g | **Saturated fat:** 3.5g | **Protein:** 11.5g | **Fiber:** 5.4g | **Sodium:** 216.2mg | **Calcium:** 69.4mg | **Potassium:** 406.5mg | **Sugar:** 2g

Tip:

Garnish with Sriracha and scallion if you want.

Ingredients:

- 1/4 avocado
- 1 slice whole-wheat bread, toasted
- 1 large egg, fried
- 1 teaspoon of Sriracha
- 1/4 teaspoon of ground pepper
- 1/8 teaspoon of garlic powder
- 1 tablespoon of scallion, sliced

Direction:

1. Combine pepper, avocado, and garlic powder in a small bowl.
2. Gently mash together.
3. Top the toast with the avocado mixture and fried egg.
4. Serve and enjoy.

A Cup Of Cottage Cheese With Peach Slices

Cook Time:

0 minutes

Prep Time:

3 minutes

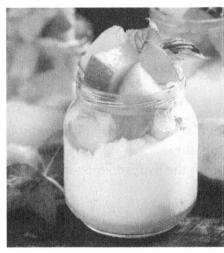

Serving Size

1

Calories per serving:

221kcal

Carbs per serving:

20g

Adding fruits is one of my favorite ways to eat cottage cheese. I love it so much! I'm sure it's a match made in heaven. It's excellent for both breakfast and lunch.

Per Serving:

Fat: 1.5g | Saturated fat: 1.5g
Protein: 29g | Fiber: 2.3g |
Sodium: 917.6mg | Calcium:
146.8mg | Potassium: 479.4mg |
Sugar: 18.7g

Tip:

You can eat cottage cheese with just about any fruit (canned in fruit juice, fresh or frozen).

Ingredients:

- 1 cup of cottage cheese, low-fat
- 1 medium raw peaches

Direction:

1. Cut the peach in half.
2. Remove pit.
3. Cut peach into bite-size pieces.
4. Mix with cottage cheese.
5. Serve yourself and enjoy it.

Peanut Butter Sandwich With Strawberry Jam

Cook Time:
0 minutes

Prep Time:
5 minutes

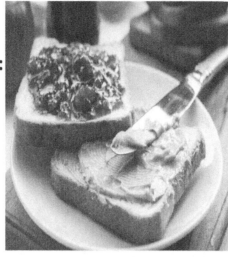

Serving Size
1
Calories per serving:
193kcal
Carbs per serving:
22g

This recipe is too creative, even for the ordinary mind. Peanut Butter Sandwich can be eaten in the morning. It's a very easy and fast sandwich. It's packed with nice flavor, and I hope you enjoy it!

Per Serving:

Fat: 83g | **Saturated fat:** 2g
Protein: 7g | **Fiber:** 2g | **Sodium:** 205.88mg | **Calcium:** 45.77mg | **Potassium:** 178.63mg | **Sugar:** 8g

Tip:

Put peanut butter on both slices of bread otherwise, the jelly can soak the bread and get your hands dirty.

Ingredients:

- 1 tablespoon of strawberry jam
- 1 tablespoon of peanut butter
- 1 slice whole-grain sandwich bread (toasted)

Direction:

1. Spread peanut butter on the sandwich first using a knife, before you add the jam.
2. Add the jam.
3. Serve and enjoy.

Chicken Nacho Casserole

Cook Time:
25 minutes

Prep Time:
5 minutes

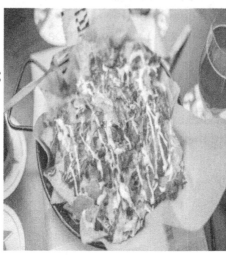

Serving Size
1
Calories
per serving:
210kcal
Carbs
per serving:
17g

Don't you believe you can have "Nachos" with diabetes? Try this healthy version that has all the flavor of traditional nachos with ZERO of all the extra carbs and fat. A good recipe that can be ready-to-eat within 30 minutes. Enjoy it!

Per Serving:

Fat: 6g | **Saturated fat:** 2.5g
Protein: 23g | **Fiber:** 3g |
Sodium: 360mg | **Calcium:** 0mg |
Potassium: 460mg | **Sugar:** 3g

Tip:

You can serve your nachos with light sour cream.

Ingredients:

- 1 nonstick cooking spray
- 2 teaspoons of chili powder
- 1/2 teaspoon of cumin
- 1/2 teaspoon of garlic powder
- 2/3 cup of cheddar cheese (reduced-fat, shredded)
- 1/8 teaspoon of black pepper
- 1 pound of chicken breasts (boneless, skinless, cut into small pieces)
- 1 can of fire-roasted tomatoes (15-ounce, diced)
- 1 cup of black beans (no salt added, drained and rinsed)
- 1-1/2 ounces of baked tortilla chips (crushed, (or about 24)

Direction:

1) Preheat the oven to 375 degrees F.
2) Use cooking spray to spray a 2-1/2 quart baking dish.
3) Season the chicken with black pepper.
4) Use cooking spray to spray a large saute pan and heat over medium-high.
5) Add the chicken. Then cook for about 8 minutes.
6) Add the black beans, diced tomatoes, chili powder, garlic powder, and cumin to the pan.
7) Reduce the heat to low. Then simmer for about 5 minutes.
8) Pour the chicken mixture into the baking dish.
9) Sprinkle cheese on top. Then top with the crushed tortilla chips.
10) Bake until the cheese is melted, for about 12 minutes.
11) Serve and enjoy.

Stir-Fried Vegetable And Egg Omelet

Cook Time:
25 minutes

Prep Time:
5 minutes

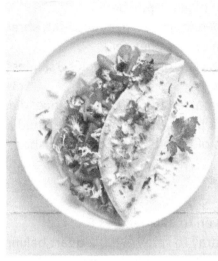

Serving Size
1

**Calories
per serving:**
128.2kcal

**Carbs
per serving:**
6.7g

This recipe is a great recipe you can eat for breakfast or dinner. If you want to enjoy this recipe, you can pair with potatoes or a slice of toast. This will even make it a complete meal. You can also add more spices to the vegetables if you want-it will still come out great! Enjoy!

Per Serving:

Tip:

Fat: 6.1g | **Saturated fat:** 1.9g
Protein: 12.3g | **Fiber:** 3.5g |
Sodium: 357.5mg | **Calcium:**
120mg | **Potassium:** 341.1mg |
Sugar: 4.1g

You can garnish with chives, if desired.

Ingredients:

- 1/2 cup of no-salt-added diced tomatoes with garlic, basil, and oregano, well-drained
- 1/2 cup of cucumber, chopped and seeded
- 1/2 cup of chopped yellow summer squash
- 1/2 ripe avocado, pitted, peeled, and chopped
- 1/4 teaspoon of ground black pepper
- 1 Nonstick cooking spray
- 1/4 cup of shredded reduced-fat Monterey Jack cheese with jalapeño chile peppers
- 2 eaches eggs
- 1 cup of refrigerated or frozen egg product, thawed
- 2 tablespoons of water
- 1 teaspoon of dried basil, crushed
- 1/4 teaspoon of salt
- 1 snipped fresh chives

Direction:

For filling:
1) Stir together cucumber, tomatoes, squash, and avocado in a medium bowl. Set it aside. Whisk together eggs, water, egg product, salt, basil, and pepper in a medium bowl.
2) For the Omelet, use cooking spray to coat an 8-inch nonstick skillet generously. Heat skillet over medium heat, and add a 1/3 cup of the egg mixture into the hot skillet.
3) Use a spatula to start stirring the eggs gently, but continuously, until the mixture resembles cooked egg pieces surrounded by liquid egg. Stop stirring, and cook until egg is set but shiny for about 30 to 60 seconds.
4) Spoon half cup of the filling over one side of the Omelet, and carefully fold Omelet over the filling. Carefully remove Omelet from the skillet and repeat to make as much Omelet you can eat. Use paper towels to wipe the skillet clean, then spray with cooking spray between omelets.
5) Sprinkle 1 tablespoon of cheese over each Omelet.
6) Serve yourself and enjoy it.

Banana And Berry Smoothie

Cook Time:
0 minutes

Prep Time:
5 minutes

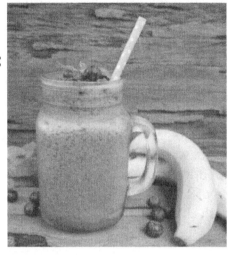

Serving Size
1
Calories per serving:
514kcal
Carbs per serving:
12g

The soft and creamy texture of the banana makes them easy to eat, and the only thing needed to get this Smoothie ready is five-minutes of your time and five ingredients to whip-up this refreshing drink. Enjoy!

Per Serving:

Fat: 24g | Unsaturated fat: 15g | Protein: 20g | Fiber: 12g | Sodium: 69mg | Sugar: 0g | Cholesterol: 10mg

Tip:

You can freeze the leftovers in an airtight, microwave container. Enjoy!

Ingredients:

- 1/2 cup of frozen blueberries
- 1 teaspoon of honey
- 1/8 teaspoon of vanilla extract
- 1/3 cup of rolled oats
- 1 tablespoon of chia seeds
- 1/2 banana
- 1/3 cup of plain Greek yogurt
- 1/3 cup of milk
- 1/4 cup of chopped walnuts, divided

Direction:

1. Place the banana, blueberries, milk, yogurt, honey, 3 tablespoons of walnuts, and vanilla in a blender.
2. Blend until smooth.
3. In a bowl, pour the blueberry-walnut mixture.
4. Stir in the chia seeds and oats.
5. Pour the mixture in a small serving container or in a jar.
6. Top with the rest of the walnuts.
7. Cover and refrigerate over the night, for about 4 hours.
8. Serve cold straight from the refrigerator.
9. Enjoy.

Made-Ahead Breakfast Quiche

Cook Time:
30 minutes

Prep Time:
15 minutes

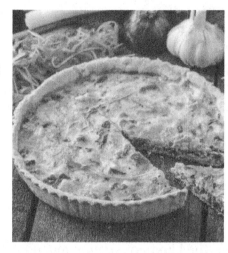

Serving Size
1
Calories per serving:
231kcal
Carbs per serving:
14g

Make-ahead Breakfast Quiche gets its creamy texture from the evaporated milk. It's a great recipe to make ahead by simply reheating before serving or cut into slices, and then reheat each morning for breakfast. Just be sure to cook the broccoli until it's just barely tender. Enjoy!

Per Serving:

Fat: 16g | Saturated fat: 8g
Protein: 10g | Fiber: 3g |
Sodium: 404mg | Calcium:
150mg | Potassium: 204mg |
Sugar: 3g

Tip:

Let edges turn golden brown for about 30 to 35 minutes and let it stand for 10 minutes just before serving.

Ingredients:

- 1 (9 inches) frozen whole-wheat pie-crust shell
- 1 (8 ounces) package of microwavable fresh broccoli florets
- 3 ounces of sharp Cheddar cheese, shredded (about 3/4 cup)
- 3/4 teaspoon of kosher salt
- 1/4 teaspoon of black pepper
- 1 1/2 teaspoons of olive oil
- 1 cup of chopped sweet onion (from 1 large onion)
- 4 large eggs large eggs
- 1/2 cup of evaporated milk

Direction:

1. Preheat oven to 400 degrees F.
2. Let the pie-crust thaw for about 10 minutes at room temperature.
3. Place in the preheated oven, and bake for about 10 to 15 minutes until lightly browned.
4. Let it cool for about 10 mins.
5. Reduce oven temperature to 375 degrees F.
6. Cook broccoli according to package instruction, for about 3 minutes, until tender-crisp. Chop larger pieces coarsely.
7. In a large skillet, heat oil over medium-high and add onion. Cook for 10 minutes, until lightly golden.
8. Whisk together evaporated milk and eggs in a medium bowl.
9. Stir in cheese, broccoli, onion, black pepper, and salt.
10. Pour mixture into prepared pie crust.
11. Bake until just set and edges are golden brown at 375 degrees F.
12. Serve and enjoy.

Cheesy Ham And Hash Casserole

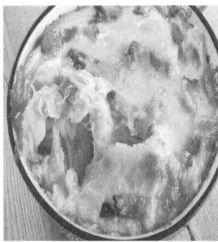

Cook Time:
1 hour

Prep Time:
15 minutes

Serving Size
1

**Calories
per serving:**
414.6kcal

**Carbs
per serving:**
29.7g

Cheesy ham and hash casserole is a quick and easy breakfast to make, not to mention delicious. It's surely going to be a hit!

Per Serving:

Fat: 27.2g | Saturated fat: 14.7g
Protein: 14.4g | Fiber: 2.4g |
Sodium: 760.6mg | Calcium:
304.1mg | Potassium: 437.8mg |
Sugar: 0.7g

Tip:

You can use 2 cans of cream of celery soup instead of cream of potato. It's still good.

Ingredients:

- 1/8 (10.75 ounces) can of condensed cream of potato soup
- 1/8 (16 ounces) container of sour cream
- 2 tablespoons and 3/4 teaspoon of shredded sharp Cheddar cheese
- 1/8 (32 ounces) package of frozen hash brown potatoes
- 1/2 ounce of cooked, diced ham
- 1 tablespoon and 1-3/4 teaspoons of grated Parmesan cheese

Direction:

1. Preheat oven to 375 degrees F.
2. Grease a 9x13-inch baking dish lightly.
3. Mix head browns, the cream of potato soup, ham, Cheddar cheese, and sour cream together in a large bowl.
4. Spread evenly into prepared dish.
5. Sprinkle with Parmesan cheese.
6. Bake for about an hour in the preheated oven, or until lightly brown and bubbly.
7. Serve immediately.
8. Enjoy.

Egg And Bacon Tacos

Cook Time:
3 minutes

Prep Time:
5 minutes

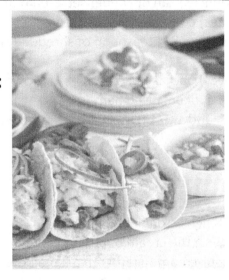

Serving Size
1
**Calories
per serving:**
435.7kcal
**Carbs
per serving:**
40.5g

This is an amazing recipe that can be served with salsa if desired. It's just a combination of some bacon and eggs on a flour tortilla, which is perfect for breakfast.

Per Serving:

Fat: 22g | Saturated fat: 9.2g
Protein: 18.9g | Fiber: 2.9g |
Sodium: 1295.4mg | Calcium:
211.7mg | Potassium: 375.4mg |
Sugar: 3.2g

Tip:

You can add a bit of onion and red pepper to this recipe if you want some veggies in it. They are in addition to the delicious flavor.

Ingredients:

- 1 egg
- 1/8 teaspoon of salt
- 1/8 teaspoon of ground black pepper
- 1 flour tortillas
- 2 teaspoons of crumbled cooked bacon
- 1 teaspoon of butter
- 1/2 slice of American cheese, diced
- 2 tablespoons and 2 teaspoons of salsa (optional)

Direction:

1) In a bowl, whisk eggs together and stir in bacon.
2) In a skillet over medium heat, melt butter and add the egg mixture.
3) Cook and stir for about 2 to 3 minutes, until eggs are completely set.
4) Stir in American cheese, pepper, and salt.
5) Wrap tortillas in damp paper towels; microwave for about a minute, until warmed through.
6) Spoon 1/8 cup of egg mixture into the center of the tortilla.
7) Fold sides to cover.
8) Serve with salsa.
9) Enjoy.

Breakfast Crepes

Cook Time:
20 minutes

Prep Time:
10 minutes

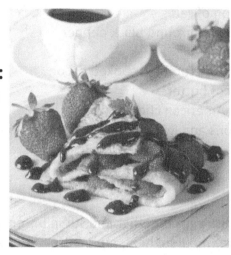

Serving Size
1

Calories per serving:
215.7kcal

Carbs per serving:
25.5g

This recipe is made with ingredients you already have in your kitchen. I hope you enjoy it!

Per Serving:

Tip:

Fat: 9.2g | **Saturated fat:** 4.9g
Protein: 7.4g | **Fiber:** 0.8g |
Sodium: 235.5mg | **Calcium:**
56.3mg | **Potassium:** 114.7mg |
Sugar: 1.7g

You can add different flavoured jams to this recipe.

Ingredients:

- 1/4 cup of all-purpose flour
- 2 tablespoons of milk
- 2 tablespoons of water
- 1/8 teaspoon of salt
- 1/2 eggs
- 1-1/2 teaspoons of butter, melted

Direction:

1. Whisk together the eggs and flour in a large mixing bowl.
2. Gradually add in the water and milk, stirring to combine.
3. Add the butter and salt; beat until smooth.
4. Bring a lightly oiled frying pan over medium-high heat.
5. Pour or scoop the batter onto the griddle, using approx—1/4 cup of each of the crepe.
6. Tilt the pan with a circular motion so the batter will coats the surface evenly.
7. Cook the crepe until the bottom is brown lightly for about 2 minutes.
8. Loosen with a spatula.
9. Turn and cook the other side.
10. Serve hot and enjoy.

No-Bake Nut Butter Protein Bites

Cook Time:
20 minutes

Prep Time:
10 minutes

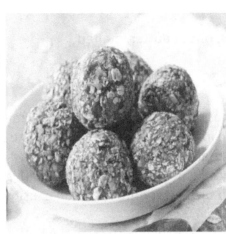

Serving Size
1
Calories per serving:
155kcal
Carbs per serving:
15g

No-Bake Nut Butter Protein Bites are the ultimate guilt-free treat loaded with old fashioned oats, flax seeds, and creamy peanut butter, sweetened to perfection with semi-sweet chocolate chips and honey. Enjoy this healthy protein-packed option that works like magic for breakfast or snack!

Per Serving:

Fat: 9g | **Saturated fat:** 2g
Protein: 4g | **Fiber:** 2g | **Sodium:** 75mg | **Calcium:** 25mg | **Potassium:** 150mg | **Sugar:** 8g

Tip:

Use a cookie scoop for the bites. It works great beacause these bites are a bit sticky to roll. Also, separate them using parchment paper if stacking in a container.

Ingredients:

- 1 cup of old fashioned oats
- 0.13 teaspoon of sea salt
- 0.5 cup of creamy peanut butter
- 0.25 cup of honey
- 0.25 cup of ground flax seed
- 1 teaspoon of vanilla extract
- 0.25 teaspoon of ground cinnamon
- 1 tablespoon of chia seeds
- 0.25 cup semi-sweet chocolate chips

Direction:

1) In a large mixing bowl, add all ingredients together, and combine.
2) Cover using plastic wrap or a lid.
3) Place the mixture inside the refrigerator for about 30 minutes (this will help in making them easier to roll)
4) Roll into your desired amount of bites using 2 tablespoons of the scooper.
5) Store in the refrigerator in an airtight container for up to 7 days. You can freeze for up to 3 months as well.
6) Serve and enjoy.

Chicken On Whole Wheat Toast With Olive Oil

Cook Time:
5 minutes

Prep Time:
5 minutes

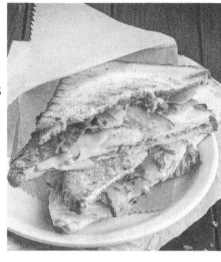

Serving Size
1
Calories per serving:
240kcal
Carbs per serving:
14g

This is a recipe with tasty warm filling, crispy bread, melty cheese that makes a satisfying, diabetes-friendly breakfast or lunch or light dinner. You can pair this recipe with a simple side salad, like avocado, spinach, and summer berry salad, for a heart-healthy and a balanced meal.
I hope you enjoy it!

Per Serving:

Fat: 9g | Saturated fat: 3g
Protein: 28g | Fiber: 2g |
Sodium: 330mg | Potassium:
250mg | Sugar: 2g

Tip:

Use a nonstick skillet that is large enough to hold the sandwich.

Ingredients:

- 1 tablespoon of light mayonnaise
- 1 slice (about 1 ounce) of crusty whole-wheat bread
- 1/4 cup fresh tarragon
- 1 piece of reduced-fat Swiss cheese
- 4 ounces cooked chicken breast
- 1/8 teaspoon of salt
- 1/8 teaspoon of black pepper
- 1/2 olive oil spray

Direction:

1. Spread mayonnaise on the bread.
2. Top with the tarragon, chicken, and cheese.
3. Sprinkle with pepper and salt, then top with rest of the slices of bread.
4. Coat a nonstick skillet with olive oil spray.
5. Heat over low heat.
6. Add the sandwich and press down using a lid or any other clean pan.
7. Cook for about 2 minutes, flip and press again. Cook for another 2 minutes.
8. Cut the sandwich into half.
9. Serve with salad and enjoy it.

Broccoli Omelet

Cook Time:
0 minutes

Prep Time:
10 minutes

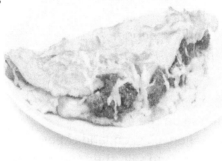

Serving Size
1
Calories
per serving:
243.7kcal
Carbs
per serving:
3.1g

The omelet is a dish of French origin, prepares with eggs cooked quickly in a pan. The broccoli and cheese omelet is a simple and tasty single dish. In a few minutes, you will prepare a good and fast dish.

Per Serving:

Fat: 20.6g | Saturated fat: 6.9g
Protein: 11.5g | Fiber: 0.6g |
Sodium: 477.8mg | Calcium:
186.2mg | Potassium: 229.6mg |
Sugar: 1.4g

Tip:

Stuff the omelet when the egg is still liquid so that the final consistency is creamy.

Ingredients:

- 2 teaspoons of extra-virgin olive oil
- 1 large egg
- 1 tablespoon of reduced-fat milk
- 2 tablespoons of shredded Monterey Jack cheese
- 1/8 teaspoon of salt
- 1/4 cup of finely chopped broccoli
- 1/4 cup of finely chopped spinach
- 1 tablespoon of reduced-fat sour cream
- 1 tablespoon of finely chopped chives

Direction:

1) Heat oil over medium heat in a small no-skillet.
2) Add spinach and broccoli, then cook, occasionally stirring, for about 2 to 4 minutes, until bright green and tender.
3) Meanwhile, whisk milk and egg in a small bowl.
4) Add the mixture into the pan, and stir to combine with the vegetables.
5) Cook, tilting the pan and letting the egg run under the edges. Cook until the egg forms a thin, even layer.
6) Continue to cook until just slightly wet, for about 2 minutes, reducing the heat if starting to brown.
7) Sprinkle with salt and cheese.
8) Roll into an omelet using a spatula.
9) Serve and enjoy.

Egg And Avocado Omelet

Cook Time:
8 minutes

Prep Time:
15 minutes

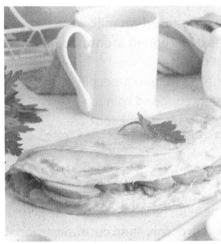

Serving Size
1
Calories
per serving:
392kcal
Carbs
per serving:
10.5g

This recipe is delicious. If you don't have feta cheese, you can use sharp cheddar as well. I doubt it will change the flavor. It's undoubtedly going to come out generous and delicious!

Per Serving:

Fat: 31.3g | Saturated fat: 12.3g
Protein: 19.1g | Fiber: 4.1g |
Sodium: 1013.6mg | Calcium:
335.9mg | Potassium: 489.6mg |
Sugar: 4.4g

Tip:

Whisk into eggs if using dried basil.

Ingredients:

- 3 large eggs eggs
- 1/4 cup of chopped kalamata olives
- 1 tablespoon of chopped fresh basil
- 3/4 cup of feta cheese
- 1/2 avocado, diced
- 1/2 cup of diced tomatoes

Direction:

1. In a small bowl, whisk eggs until smooth.
2. Preheat a nonstick skillet over medium heat.
3. Pour in eggs and scatter avocado, feta cheese, olives, tomatoes, and basil over 1 side.
4. Cook for about 5 minutes until the bottom is golden brown.
5. Fold over; cook for about 3 minutes, until center is set.
6. Serve and enjoy.

Apple And Cinnamon Overnight Oats

Cook Time:
0 minutes

Prep Time:
10 minutes

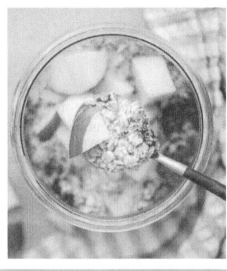

Serving Size
1
Calories per serving:
215.3kcal
Carbs per serving:
40.8g

Apple and Cinnamon Overnight Oats takes a few minutes in the evening to mix almond milk and rolled oats together, and you have a head start on a healthy breakfast the following morning. Then in the morning, you can just top the oatmeal with toasted nuts and fresh fruits - *so great!*

Per Serving:

Fat: 4.4g | **Saturated fat:** 0.5g
Protein: 5.8g | **Fiber:** 6.3g |
Sodium: 231.8mg | **Calcium:**
262mg | **Potassium:** 248.9mg |
Sugar: 11.3g

Tip:

Use oats "gluten-free" oats, as oats often cross-contaminated with barley and wheat.

Ingredients:

- 1/2 cup of old-fashioned rolled oats
- 1/4 teaspoon of ground cinnamon
- 1 pinch of salt
- 1/2 cup of diced apple
- 1/2 cup of unsweetened almond milk
- 1/2 tablespoon of chia seeds
- 1 teaspoon of maple syrup
- 2 tablespoons of toasted pecans

Direction:

1) Combine almond milk, oats, chia seeds (if using), cinnamon, maple syrup, and salt in a pint-sized jar.
2) Stir together.
3) Cover and refrigerate over the night.
4) Before serving, top with pecans and apple, if you feel like.
5) Serve and enjoy.

Egg Muffins

Cook Time:
10 minutes

Prep Time:
25 minutes

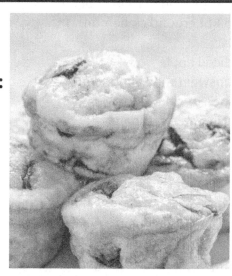

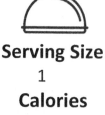

Serving Size
1

Calories per serving:
50kcal

Carbs per serving:
1g

These egg muffins are low-carb and diabetic friendly as well. They are a simple breakfast, great for meal prepping. They store well in the fridge for up to 7 days, or you can freeze them and store for up to 3 months. You would love this muffin!

Per Serving:

Fat: 3g | **Saturated fat:** 1g
Protein: 6g | **Fiber:** 1g | **Sodium:** 135mg | **Potassium:** 105mg | **Sugar:** 0g

Tip:

You can freeze the muffins and store in a freezer bag for up to 3 months.

Ingredients:

- 1 nonstick cooking spray
- 1/2 cup of thawed and squeezed frozen chopped spinach
- 2 eggs
- 1 egg whites
- 1/8 cup of plain nonfat Greek yogurt
- 1/8 teaspoon of salt
- 1/8 teaspoon of black pepper
- 1/8 cup of grated Parmesan cheese

Direction:

1) Preheat the oven to 350 degrees F.
2) Spray each cup of the muffin pan using 1 spray of non-stick cooking spray.
3) Add 1 heaping tablespoon of thawed spinach into the bottom of each muffin cup inside the muffin tin.
4) Whisk together the eggs, egg whites, salt, yogurt, and pepper in a medium bowl.
5) Place the egg mixture into the muffin cups.
6) Top each of the egg muffins with 1 teaspoon of Parmesan cheese and place in the oven, then bake until the eggs are slightly firm to touch, for about 20 to 25 min.
7) Remove from the oven. Cool by setting it aside, for about 5 mins.
8) Remove muffins from the pan and serve or store in the refrigerator in an airtight container.
9) Place the muffin on a plate uncovered in the microwave for some seconds to reheat from the refrigerator.
10) Serve and enjoy.

Blueberry And Nuts Overnight Oats

Cook Time:
0 minutes

Prep Time:
5 minutes

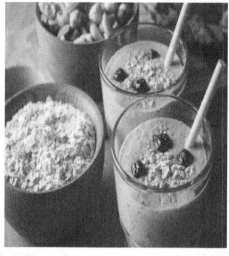

Serving Size
1
**Calories
per serving:**
514kcal
**Carbs
per serving:**
12g

Blueberry and nuts overnight oats would be the winner if there was a prize for the breakfast that delivers the highest reward for the least amount of effort. You only stir some ingredients together, let them mix and mingle in the fridge while you sleep. Wake up in the morning, and you have a satisfying breakfast all ready to go.

Per Serving:

Fat: 24g | **Unsaturated fat:** 15g | **Protein:** 20g | **Fiber:** 12g | **Sodium:** 69mg | **Sugar:** 0g | **Cholesterol:** 10mg

Tip:

Serve cold straight from the refrigerator, and enjoy!

Ingredients:

- 1/2 cup of frozen blueberries
- 1 teaspoon of honey
- 1/8 teaspoon of vanilla extract
- 1/3 cup of rolled oats
- 1 tablespoon of chia seeds
- 1/2 banana
- 1/3 cup of plain Greek yogurt
- 1/3 cup of milk
- 1/4 cup of chopped walnuts, divided

Direction:

1. Place the banana, blueberries, milk, yogurt, honey, 3 tablespoons of walnuts, and vanilla in a blender.
2. Blend until smooth.
3. In a bowl, pour the blueberry-walnut mixture.
4. Stir in the chia seeds and oats.
5. Pour the mixture in a small serving container or in a jar.
6. Top with the rest of the walnuts.
7. Cover and refrigerate over the night, for about 4 hours.
8. Serve cold straight from the refrigerator.
9. Enjoy.

Apple And Cinnamon Pancakes

Cook Time:
1 hour

Prep Time:
15 minutes

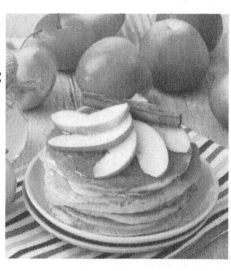

Serving Size
1

Calories per serving:
176.1kcal

Carbs per serving:
27.5g

Apple and Cinnamon Pancakes use 100% whole-wheat flour, a tablespoon of added sugar, and heart-healthy canola oil. If you want to experiment with several types of whole grains, you can replace up to 1/2 cup of the flour with cornmeal, oats, or buckwheat flour.

Per Serving:

Fat: 5.2g | **Saturated fat:** 0.8g
Protein: 6.2g | **Fiber:** 3.4g |
Sodium: 377.6mg | **Calcium:**
147.5mg | **Potassium:** 154mg |
Sugar: 7.1g

Tip:

Resist over-mixing the wet and dry ingredients, so the pancake won't be tough.

Ingredients:

- 1/2 cup of white whole-wheat flour
- 1 teaspoon of baking powder
- 1/2 cup of buttermilk
- 1/2 cup of grated apple
- 1 tablespoon of canola oil
- 1/2 tablespoon of sugar
- 1/2 teaspoon of vanilla extract
- 1/2 teaspoon of ground cinnamon
- 1/8 teaspoon of baking soda
- 1/8 teaspoon of salt
- 1 large egg

Direction:

1) Whisk baking powder, flour, baking soda, cinnamon, and salt in a large bowl.
2) Whisk buttermilk, egg, apple, sugar, oil, and vanilla in a medium bowl.
3) In the center of the dry ingredients, make a well, add the wet ingredients, and whisk until combined.
4) Let batter sir, for about 10 minutes, without stirring.
5) The baking powder forms bubbles that create fluffy pancakes as the batter rests and the gluten in the flour relaxes to make them more tender.
6) Use cooking spray to coat a large nonstick skillet; heat over medium heat.
7) Measure out pancakes using about 1/8 cup of batter per pancake, without stirring the batter, and pout into the pan.
8) Cook until you see bubbles on the surface, and the edges are dry.
9) Repeat with the remaining batter, using cooking spray to coat the pan.
10) Reduce the heat as needed.
11) Serve and enjoy.

Quesadilla

Cook Time:
16 minutes

Prep Time:
15 minutes

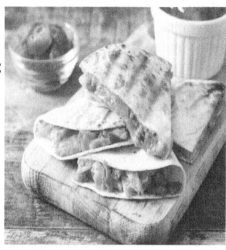

Serving Size
1

Calories per serving:
160kcal

Carbs per serving:
8g

Quesadillas are made with spicy chiles and fluffy eggs folded into a tortilla with rich melted cheese, which makes breakfast a pleasure! You can use a variety of cheese, such as Monterey Jack, white cheddar, and asadero.

Per Serving:

Fat: 10g | **Saturated fat:** 4g
Protein: 14g | **Fiber:** 5g |
Sodium: 460mg | **Calcium:** 0mg |
Potassium: 135mg | **Sugar:** 1g

Tip:

Serve your Quesadilla immediately with salsa. Refrigerate the leftovers. They can be refrigerated in an airtight container for up to 4 days.

Ingredients:

- 1 nonstick cooking spray
- 2 10-inch whole wheat flour tortillas
- 1-1/2 cup of reduced-fat cheddar cheese, or use Mexican blend, Monterey Jack, or pepper jack (reduced fat)
- 1/4 cup of canned green chiles
- 4 eggs (beaten)
- 1/4 teaspoon of black pepper
- 4 slice of turkey bacon (cooked crisp and crumbled)

Direction:

1. Use cooking spray to coat a small skillet lightly.
2. Saute green chiles over medium-low heat for about 2 minutes.
3. Add the beaten eggs, and cook. Stir until scrambled and set.
4. Season with pepper.
5. Use cooking spray to coat a second large skillet lightly.
6. Place one tortilla in the skillet. Then cook over medium-heat until air bubbles start to form, for about 1 minute.
7. Flip the tortilla over and cook for about 1 minute - don't let the tortilla get crispy here.
8. Spread half of the cheese evenly over the tortilla, but covering to the edges.
9. Reduce the heat to low and quickly arrange half of the cooked bacon with half of the egg mixture over the cheese.
10. Cook for about 1 minute, until the cheese starts to melt.
11. Fold the tortilla in half to create a half-moon shape.
12. Flip folded tortilla over and cook until the cheese filling is completely melted and lightly toasted, for about 2 minutes.
13. Transfer the quesadilla to a cutting board. Use cooking spray to recoat the skillet and repeat with the second tortilla and the rest of the bacon, egg mixture, and cheese.
14. Cut each of the quesadillas into 3 wedges.
15. Serve immediately with fresh salsa and enjoy.

Lunch
Recipes

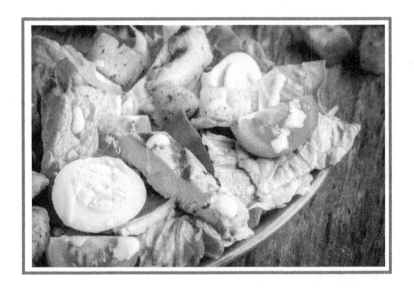

Spinach Rolls

Cook Time:
40 minutes

Prep Time:
15 minutes

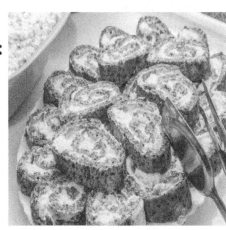

Serving Size
1

Calories per serving:
310kcal

Carbs per serving:
19.6g

These healthy spinach rolls are perfect and easy for meal prep. They are filling, savory, and have just a touch of spice for a delicious meal you can eat on the go. They only take about 15 minutes to prep, and this recipe has just a few steps to come together; each one is very straightforward, and the result is topnotch!

Per Serving:

Fat: 10.4g | **Saturated fat:** 4.6g
Protein: 27.3g | **Fiber:** 5.1g |
Sodium: 695mg | **Calcium:**
419mg | **Potassium:** 2489.3mg |
Sugar: 6.7g

Tip:

Store them in an airtight container for up to 3 to 4 days in the refrigerator.

Ingredients:

- 8 ounces of frozen spinach leaves
- 1.5 eggs
- 0.5 teaspoon of curry powder
- 0.13 teaspoon of chili flakes
- 0.5 teaspoon of salt
- 0.5 teaspoon of pepper
- 1.25 ounces of onion
- 1 ounce of carrot
- 0.5 ounce of low-fat mozzarella cheese
- 2 ounces of fat-free cottage cheese
- 0.38 cup of parsley
- 0.5 cloves garlic
- Cooking spray

Direction:

1. Preheat oven to 400 degrees F.
2. Thaw the spinach and use a strainer to squeeze out the water.
3. Mix 2 eggs, the spinach, garlic, mozzarella, pepper, and half the salt in a mixing bowl.
4. Place parchment paper on a baking sheet, and spray using cooking spray.
5. Transfer the spinach mixture to the sheet, and press it flat.
6. Bake for about 15 minutes, then set it aside to cool on a rack. Do not turn off the oven.
7. Chop parsley and onion finely. Grate the carrots.
8. Fry the onions for 1-min in a skillet with a little cooking spray. Then add the parsley and carrots to the pan and let it simmer for about 2 minutes.
9. Add curry, cottage cheese, chili, pepper, and the other half of the salt.
10. Mix briefly, and take the skillet off the heat. Add an egg and mix it all together.
11. Spread the filling just over the spinach. Don't spread it all the way to the corners, so it won't spill out when you roll it up.

12. Roll up the spinach mat and filling carefully, then bake for about 25 minutes.
13. Take out the roll once the time is up and let it cool before cutting it into slices and serving for about 5 to 10 minutes.
14. Serve and enjoy.

Smoked Salmon Wrap

Cook Time:

0 minute

Prep Time:

7 minutes

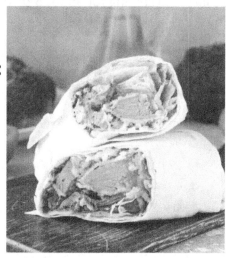

Serving Size

1

Calories per serving:

90kcal

Carbs per serving:

12g

Smoked salmon wraps are incredibly delicious and come out together in just a few minutes! It! It's so quick and easy to make, and it's such a great lunch wrap that will have you out the door in no time!

Per Serving:

Fat: 4.5g | **Saturated fat:** 1.3g
Protein: 8g | **Fiber:** 7g | **Sodium:** 465mg| **Potassium:** 140mg | **Sugar:** 1g

Tip:

You can serve with lemon wedges if you want.

Ingredients:

- 2 1/2 tablespoons of light cream cheese spread
- 1 small zucchini, trimmed
- 4 whole wheat flour tortillas (6 to 7 inches in diameter), low-carb
- 1 1/2 ounces of thinly sliced smoked salmon, cut into strips
- 2 teaspoons of snipped fresh chives
- 1 teaspoon of finely shredded lemon peel
- 2 tablespoons of lemon juice
- Lemon wedges (optional)

Direction:

1) Combine the cream cheese spread, lemon peel, chives, and lemon juice in a small bowl, stirring until smooth; set it aside.
2) Draw and make a sharp vegetable peeler along the zucchini, to cut very thin ribbons.
3) Spread the cream cheese mixture evenly over the tortillas, leaving a half-inch border around the edges.
4) Divide the salmon among the tortillas, placing it on one-half of each tortilla.
5) Layer the zucchini ribbons on the salmon.
6) Starting from the filled side, roll up the tortillas.
7) Cut each wrap into halves.
8) Serve and enjoy.

Chicken And Egg Salad Bowl

Cook Time:
20 minutes

Prep Time:
5 minutes

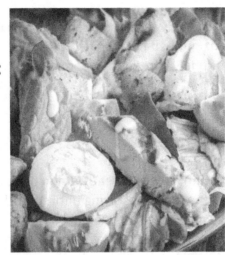

Serving Size
1
Calories per serving:
175kcal
Carbs per serving:
1.6g

This recipe is amazing, super easy to put togheter, and is perfect for meal prepping. You can make a huge batch of this delicious meal in just 25 minutes!

Per Serving:

Fat: 5.4g | **Saturated fat:** 1.1g
Protein: 30.4g | **Fiber:** 0.8g |
Sodium: 152.7mg | **Calcium:**
48mg | **Potassium:** 65.9mg |
Sugar: 0.7g

Tip:

Chilling your salad in the fridge over the night will deepen and intensify the flavor.

Ingredients:

- 0.5 tablespoon of fat-free mayo
- 0.25 tablespoon of curry powder
- 0.5 cooked chicken breasts
- 0.75 hard-boiled eggs
- Chives or basil (optional)
- Salt (optional)

Direction:

1. Bake the chicken in the oven at 365 degrees F for about 20 minutes. Make sure you check with a knife to know if the chicken is cooked all the way through.
2. Boil the eggs for about 8 minutes.
3. Cut the eggs and chicken into bite-sized pieces.
4. Mix the mayonnaise with curry powder.
5. Combine everything in a large bowl. Then mix.
6. Allow chilling in the fridge for at least 10 minutes. You can leave it in the fridge overnight if it gets better.
7. Serve on toast or muffins with a little salt and chives on top.
8. Enjoy.

Spicy Chicken Sandwich

Cook Time:
0 minutes

Prep Time:
10 minutes

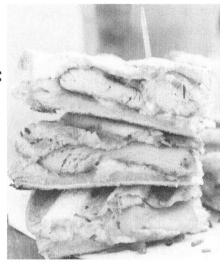

Serving Size
1

Calories per serving:
325.8kcal

Carbs per serving:
17.8g

Spicy Chicken Sandwich is a lunch recipe you will absolutely love. The Greek Yogurt takes the place of mayonnaise in this healthy sandwich, and it's fantastic. You'll love this!

Per Serving:

Fat: 19.4g | **Saturated fat:** 3.3g
Protein: 21.4g | **Fiber:** 3.2g |
Sodium: 305.7mg | **Calcium:**
88.8mg | **Potassium:** 329.2mg |
Sugar: 4.4g

Tip:

Garnish your chicken sandwich with cilantro, if you want. Enjoy!

Ingredients:

- 2 ounces (1/2 can) of canned chicken in water, drained
- 1 tablespoon of low-fat plain Greek yogurt
- 1/4 teaspoon of curry powder
- 1/8 teaspoon of ground cumin
- 1/8 teaspoon of salt
- 1/8 teaspoon of pepper
- 1 slice 100% whole-wheat bread
- 1 tablespoon of olive oil
- 4 eaches raisins, chopped
- 2 almonds or cashews, chopped
- 1/4 cup of shredded carrot
- 1 bunch of fresh cilantro

Direction:

1) In a small bowl, combine yogurt, chicken, raisins, oil, carrot, almonds (or cashews), curry powder, salt, cumin (if using), and pepper in a small bowl.
2) Lightly toast bread, if you want.
3) Spread the chicken mixture on the bread.
4) Serve and enjoy.

Greek Yogurt With Apple And Cinnamon

Cook Time:
20 minutes

Prep Time:
10 minutes

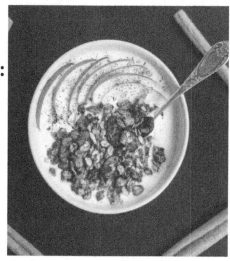

Serving Size
1

Calories per serving:
283kcal

Carbs per serving:
40g

Greek Yogurt With Apple and Cinnamon is like having apple pie for lunch, without the crust! Yogurt bowls are easy and make the perfect blank canvas for anything you're topping them with. They are a deliciously healthy fall treat you need to try for lunch today!

Per Serving:

Fat: 10g | Saturated fat: 1g
Protein: 12.5g | Fiber: 3g |
Sodium: 161mg | Sugar: 31.5g

Tip:

For make ahead, refrigerate them in a separate bowl if you want to prepare the apples in advance. Then add along with the nuts just before serving.

Ingredients:

- 1/2 sweet apple, cored, seeded, peeled, and diced (Honey Crisp, Gala)
- pinch of nutmeg
- 1 cup 0% fat of plain yogurt
- 2 tablespoons of chopped pecans or walnuts
- 1 tablespoon of raw sugar
- 1/2 tablespoon of golden raisins
- 1/8 teaspoon of cinnamon

Direction:

1. Place sugar, the diced apple, and raisins in a small pot.
2. Add water, 1/4 cup of water.
3. Sprinkle with a pinch of nutmeg and cinnamon.
4. Cover and cook over low heat for about 16 to 18 minutes, until soft.
5. Set it aside to cool.
6. Place the yogurt in the bowl.
7. Top with apples and chopped nuts.
8. Serve immediately, and enjoy.

Chicken Salad Bowl With Olive Oil Dressing

Cook Time:
20 minutes

Prep Time:
10 minutes

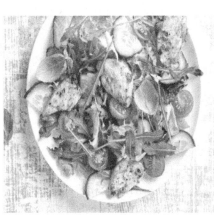

Serving Size
1

Calories per serving:
273kcal

Carbs per serving:
5g

You need to try this Chicken Salad Bowl With Olive Oil Dressing if you're not a fan of celery and mayonnaise in your chicken salad. It's made with olive oil, and it's extremely delicious!

Per Serving:

Fat: 15g | **Saturated fat:** 4g
Protein: 29g | **Fiber:** 2g |
Sodium: 734mg | **Sugar:** 3g

Tip:

For the serving, you can mix the salad into the lettuce as well.

Ingredients:

- 0.5 tablespoons of olive oil extra virgin
- 0.25 tablespoon of red wine vinegar
- 0.5 cooked chicken breasts medium, cubed
- 0.06 cup of feta crumbled
- 0.06 cup of cilantro chopped
- 1.5 cups of lettuce shredded
- 0.13 teaspoon of Diamond Crystal kosher salt
- 0.06 teaspoon of black pepper freshly ground
- 0.06 cup of red onion minced
- 0.13 cup of olives pitted, green or black (or a mix)

Direction:

Preparing the dressing:

1) Mix the olive oil, black pepper vinegar, and salt in a large bowl.
2) Add the olives, onions, chicken, cilantro, and feta into the bowl with the dressing.
3) Gently toss to combine.
4) Serve on a bed of shredded lettuce.
5) Enjoy.

Spicy Pork On A Whole Wheat Roll

Cook Time:
30 minutes

Prep Time:
30 minutes

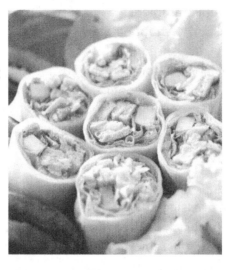

Serving Size
1

Calories per serving:
314kcal

Carbs per serving:
17.8g

The spicy pork in this recipe takes the roll game to another level, like Whoa. You can make a roll if you can make a burrito, and personally, I find that rice paper more forgiving than tortillas.

Per Serving:

Fat: 13.4g | **Protein:** 9.9g | **Sodium:** 1083.2mg | **Sugar:** 9.7g

Tip:

You can add some Asian noodles to the roll and doused the inside with the dipping sauce.

Ingredients:

- 1 cucumber, sliced and peeled thin
- 1 handful of basil, julienned
- Lettuce
- 1 pound of marinated boneless pork chops
- 1 red pepper, sliced very thin
- Rice Papers for rolling
- (Note: You can add tons of things to these rolls like other herbs, bean sprouts, etc.)

Marinade:
- 3 cloves garlic, minced
- 2 tablespoons of soy sauce (gluten-free)
- 1 teaspoon of brown sugar
- 2 tablespoons of sesame oil
- 1 shallot, minced
- 2 Thai chilies, diced (or a jalapeno)
- 1 tablespoon of fish sauce
- 2 teaspoons of freshly ground black pepper

Dipping sauce:
- 2 cloves garlic, crushed
- 1 tablespoon of rice vinegar
- 1 tablespoon of sriracha
- 1/2 cup of hoisin sauce (gluten-free)
- 1/4 cup of smooth peanut butter

Direction:

For marinade:
1. Add all ingredients in a bowl, then add pork chops in a plastic bag with marinade. Let it sit for at least 1 hour.
2. Grill on high heat or cook in a cast-iron skillet to cook the pork chops for about 4 to 5 minutes per side depending on pork chop's thickness.

3. Let it rest before slicing into them, for about 10 minutes. Slice them thinly.
4. Prep all over the veggies for rolls, and be sure to spend time slicing evenly and thinly.

For the dipping sauce:
5. Add all ingredients in a food processor. Pulse for some time to combine (you can just mix everything really well in a bowl if you don't have a food processor).

Making the rolls:
6. Start by pouring some warm water into a large plate.
7. Add a spring roll wrapper into the plate and flip it over once or maybe twice until it becomes flexible and relaxes, probably about 15 to 20 seconds.
8. Move wrapper into a clean work-surface.
9. Add some strips of pork along with some strips of all other veggies to the wrapper - make sure you don't add the fillings to the middle of the wrapper.
10. Fold the wrapper over the filling, staying away from you, then fold the edges in, and go ahead with making the rolls.
11. Pull back on the filling as you roll. This will help keep it tight and snug in the wrapper.
12. Slice them in half once you have all the rolls wrapped.
13. Serve them with the sauce and enjoy it.

Green Salad With Creamy Dressing

Cook Time:
0 minute

Prep Time:
5 minutes

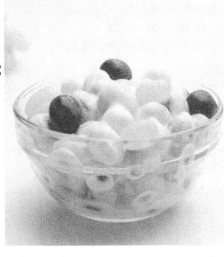

Serving Size
1

Calories per serving:
57kcal

Carbs per serving:
12.7g

You need to tickle your taste buds with this medley of grapes and green veggies, tossed in a creamy yet low-fat sour and sweet dressing. The dressing features low-fat curds laced with a streak of spices and honey, which gives the salad a luscious and rich, refreshing, and mouth feeling taste despite the low-calorie count.

Per Serving:

Fat: 0.2g | Protein: 1.4g | Fiber: 1.6g | Sodium: 113.2mg | Sugar: 0g

Tip:

You can pair this salad with a soup like pumpkin soup.

Ingredients:

- 1/4 cup of cucumber cubes
- 1/4 cup of seedless grapes
- 1/8 cup of capsicum cubes
- 1/4 tablespoon of honey
- 1/8 cup of fresh, low-fat curds
- freshly ground black pepper, to taste
- salt
- 1/4 teaspoons of mustard powder (Sarson/rai)

Direction:

1) In a small bowl, combine all the salad ingredients.
2) Pour the dressing over it, and toss it well.
3) Refrigerate for at least 1 hour.
4) Serve chilled, and enjoy.

A Cup Of Greek Yogurt With Berries And Chia Seeds

Cook Time:
0 minute

Prep Time:
1 minute

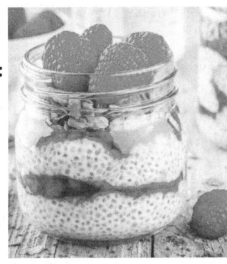

Serving Size
1

Calories per serving:
42kcal

Carbs per serving:
3.9g

Enjoy a cup of Greek Yogurt with Berries and Chia Seeds for lunch. All you need to do is put milk, yogurt, and chia seeds in a bowl, give it a stir and place it in the refrigerator. After some hours, the chia seeds
till transform into a nourishing lunch.
I hope you enjoy this quick lunch.

Per Serving:

Fat: 2g | Saturated fat: 1.1g
Protein: 2.1g | Fiber: 0.6g |
Sodium: 25mg | Calcium: 71mg |
Potassium: 102mg | Sugar: 3.6g

Tip:

You can use the empty glass container to save time on measuring the milk. The amount of milk will just be about a full jar of milk.

Ingredients:

- 1 tablespoon of chia seeds
- 1/2 handful chocolate granola (use your favorite brand)
- 1/2 handful raspberries
- 0.25 cup of raspberry yogurt (you can use Glenilen Farm Raspberry Yogurt)
- 0.25 cup of whole milk
- additional yogurt - for topping (if desired) (you can use a plain yogurt if you want to reduce the total amount of sugar)

Direction:

1. In a medium bowl, add yogurt and milk together, and combine.
2. Stir in the chia seeds. Cover, and set in the refrigerator over the night.
3. Stir the chia-seed mixture several times after putting it in the refrigerator, if you can, for about 30 to 60 minutes. It will help in preventing clumps.
4. Give the chia-seed pudding a good mix, breaking apart any clumps.
5. Stir in an extra spoonful or two of the yogurt, if you feel like.
6. Spoon into bowls or into the reserved yogurt container.
7. Top with some fresh raspberries and chocolate granola.
8. Serve yourself and enjoy it.

A Cup Of Cottage Cheese With Olive Oil And Diced Cherry Tomatoes

Cook Time:
0 minute

Prep Time:
45 minutes

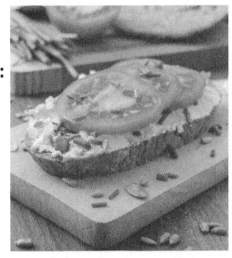

Serving Size
1

Calories per serving:
49kcal

Carbs per serving:
2.9g

You can go to the farmers market, pick up some fresh tomatoes, make this topping with any hot sauce, and then top it with some minced chives. You would love it because it's so easy and straightforward to prepare. I hope you enjoy eating this for lunch.

Per Serving:

Fat: 3.2g |
Protein: 3.8g | **Fiber:** 1.4g |
Sodium: 0mg | **Calcium:** 0mg |
Potassium: 0mg | **Sugar:** 1.1g

Tip:

Season with lots of black pepper and salt before serving.

Ingredients:

- Baguette (or any bread you have around)
- Good quality Extra-Virgin Olive Oil
- Chives; chopped
- Cottage cheese
- Sweet cherry tomatoes; sliced thinly
- Salt and freshly ground pepper

Direction:

1) Toast baguette or the other bread.
2) Spread some cottage cheese on top.
3) Top it with some slices of the cherry tomatoes.
4) Sprinkle with chives.
5) Drizzle with olive oil.
6) Serve and enjoy.

Chicken And Salad Wrap

Cook Time:
30 minute

Prep Time:
10 minutes

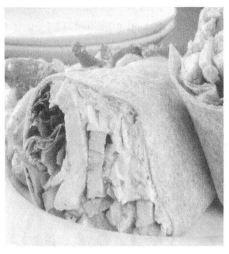

Serving Size
1

Calories per serving:
406.1kcal

Carbs per serving:
43.7g

Chicken and Salad Wraps are guaranteed crowd-pleasers. They are perfect for any leftover grilled chicken, and the distinctive salty flavor from the fish sauce
is balanced by lemon juice and fresh mint.
Enjoy!

Per Serving:

Fat: 7.7g | **Saturated fat:** 2g
Protein: 39.5g | **Fiber:** 4.6g |
Sodium: 1147.7mg | **Calcium:**
146.6mg | **Potassium:** 769.9mg |
Sugar: 10.1g

Tip:

Stack between two damp paper towels to warm tortillas in a microwave until heated through or for about 30 to 60 seconds on high.

Ingredients:

- 8 eaches 6-inch flour tortillas
- 4 cups of shredded romaine lettuce
- 3 cups of shredded cooked chicken, (12 ounces)
- 1 large tomato (cut into thin wedges)
- 1 cup of grated carrots, (2 medium)
- 1/2 cup of lemon juice
- 1/3 cup of fish sauce
- 1/4 cup of sugar
- 2 cloves garlic, minced
- 1/4 teaspoon of crushed red pepper
- 2/3 cup of chopped scallions, (1 bunch)
- 2/3 cup of slivered fresh mint

Direction:

1. Whisk fish sauce, lemon juice, garlic, sugar, and crushed red pepper in a small bowl until sugar is dissolved.
2. Preheat oven to 325 degrees F.
3. Wrap tortillas in foil and heat in the oven until softened and heated through, for about 10 to 15 minutes. Keep warm.
4. Combine chicken, lettuce, carrots, tomato, mint, and scallions in a large bowl.
5. Add 1/3 cup of the dressing and toss to coat.
6. Set out the tortillas, chicken mixture, and the rest of the dressing to assemble wraps at the table.
7. Serve immediately and enjoy it.

Apple And Cottage Cheese Salad

Cook Time:
0 minute

Prep Time:
10 minutes

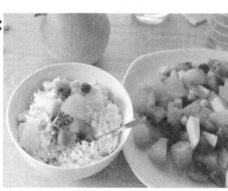

Serving Size
1

Calories per serving:
100kcal

Carbs per serving:
36.1g

A great way to shed some extra carbs off your body is having this Apple And Cottage Cheese Salad for lunch. This recipe is full of palatable flavors that are loaded with essential nutrients you need for the body. Making this recipe can be pulled off by anyone and is an easy task.

Per Serving:

Fat: 8.1g | **Saturated fat:** 1.4g
Protein: 4.8g | **Fiber:** 5.7g |
Sodium: 702mg | **Calcium:** 32mg
| **Potassium:** 332mg | **Sugar:** 26.5g

Tip:

Just before serving, add the crumbled cottage cheese carefully with raisins in the mixture. Then toss well and serve.

Ingredients:

- 2 tablespoons of cottage cheese
- 1/2 tablespoon of extra-virgin olive oil
- 1/2 cabbage red
- 1/4 cup of arugula
- 1/2 teaspoon of apple cider
- 1/2 tablespoon of lemon juice
- 1/2 tablespoon of raisins
- black pepper as required
- 1 apple
- 1/4 teaspoon of salt

Direction:

1) Wash and peel the apples. Then chop them on a chopping board into cubes.
2) Also, chop the arugula and red cabbage separately.
3) Crumble the cottage cheese using a spoon or your clean hands.
4) Take a deep bottomed bowl and add the chopped cabbage, apples, and arugula.
5) Use a wooden spoon to mix all ingredients together.
6) Pour extra virgin olive oil to the chopped fruits followed by lemon juice, apple cider vinegar, salt, and pepper.
7) Inside the bowl, mix all the ingredients thoroughly.
8) Serve and enjoy.

Hummus And Green Salad

Cook Time:
0 minute

Prep Time:
10 minutes

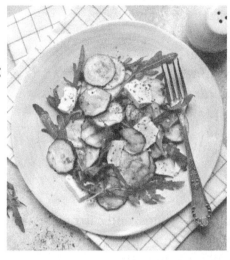

Serving Size
1

Calories per serving:
373.5kcal

Carbs per serving:
52.6g

You'll enjoy the oil and balsamic vinegar dressing of this recipe. It's such a great lunch. The dressing will make the salad taste very fresh, and you'll find this meal very filling. The hummus and pita bread (if using) is a real treat, and they are one of my go-to snacks for lunch. I hope you love it too!

Per Serving:

Fat: 14.5g | **Saturated fat:** 2g
Protein: 13.5g | **Fiber:** 10.7g |
Sodium: 795.8mg | **Calcium:**
109.4mg | **Potassium:** 732.1mg |
Sugar: 5.3g

Tip

Serve with hummus and pita.

Ingredients:

- 2 cups of mixed salad greens
- 1/2 cup of sliced cucumber
- 1 pinch of salt
- 1 pinch of ground pepper
- 1 -6 1/2-inch of whole-wheat pita bread, toasted
- 1/4 cup of hummus
- 2 tablespoons of grated carrot
- 1 -1/2 teaspoons of extra-virgin olive oil
- 1 -1/2 teaspoons of balsamic vinegar

Direction:

1. Arrange cucumber, greens, and carrots on a large plate.
2. Drizzle with vinegar and oil.
3. Sprinkle with pepper and salt.
4. Serve and enjoy.

Chicken Cauliflower Salad Bowl

Cook Time:
30 minute

Prep Time:
15 minutes

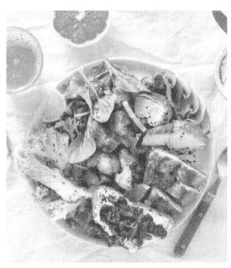

Serving Size
1

Calories per serving:
332kcal

Carbs per serving:
24g

If you're a lover of chicken, then this warm and satisfying lunch salad will be perfect for you any time of the year.

Per Serving:

Fat: 13g | Saturated fat: 2.5g
Protein: 32g | Fiber: 8| Sodium: 652mg | Calcium: 20% DV | Potassium: 296mg | Sugar: 3.5g

Tip:

You can top Salad with sliced chicken.

Ingredients:

- 1/8 cup of balsamic vinegar
- 1 teaspoon of Dijon mustard
- 1 teaspoon of honey
- 1 teaspoon of salt, divided
- 0.25 teaspoon of pepper
- 1-1/2 tablespoons of olive oil
- 2 cloves garlic
- 2 boneless, skinless chicken breasts
- 2 cups of small cauliflower florets
- 1/2 can of cannelloni beans, drained and rinsed
- 1/8 cup of Parmesan cheese, shredded
- 2 cups of baby spinach leaves
- 1/2 cup of roasted red pepper, thinly sliced
- 0.25 cup of onion, thinly sliced

Direction:

1) Preheat the oven to 425 degrees F. Line a large baking sheet with foil. Grease well and set it aside. Whisk the vinegar with the honey, pepper, mustard, and salt. Drizzle in the oil slowly while constantly whisking - do this until the mixture comes together.
2) Measure out 1/8 cup, and set it aside. Stir garlic into the rest of the mixture. Toss the chicken with 1/2 tablespoon of the garlic mixture—season all over with the rest of the salt.
3) Arrange on the prepared pan, and toss the cauliflower with the rest of the garlic mixture. In a single layer, spread on the same pan next to the chicken. Bake until a meat thermometer reads 165 degrees F, for about 20 to 25 minutes, when inserted in the center of the largest chicken breast. Transfer chicken to a cutting board. Tent with foil. Sprinkle Parmesan and beans over cauliflower.
4) Roast until browned, or for 10 minutes, and slightly cool.
5) Meanwhile, thinly slice each chicken breast and set it aside.
6) Toss cauliflower mixture with red pepper, spinach, reserved dressing, and red onion. Serve immediately and enjoy it.

Slow Cooker Vegetable Soup With Whole Wheat Toast

Cook Time:
8 hours

Prep Time:
20 minutes

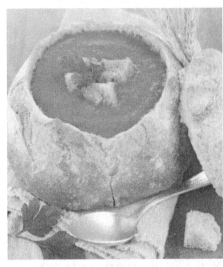

Serving Size
1

Calories per serving:
768kcal

Carbs per serving:
0g

This soup is delicious. Imagine having this perfect comfort food for lunch and dinner. The day you prepare this recipe will definitely be a great day.
It's amazing.

Per Serving:

Fat: 39g | Saturated fat: 21g
Protein: 27g | Fiber: 7g |
Sodium: 1401mg | Sugar: 13g

Tip:

Cut off the top portion of the bread, then hollow out the bowl carefully, leaving a 1/4-inch shell. Fill the bowl with soup.

Ingredients:

For the Soup:
- 1 can diced tomato with garlic & oregano & basil
- 1/4 cup of butter
- 1/4 cup of all-purpose flour
- 1/2 cup of Parmesan cheese
- 1 cup of half & half
- 1 stalk celery, finely chopped
- 1-1/2 medium carrots, finely chopped
- 1/2 small onion, finely chopped
- 1 teaspoon of Italian seasoning
- 1/2 carton of chicken broth or vegetable

- Salt and pepper, to taste

For the Bread Bowls:
- 1 tablespoon of olive oil
- 1/4 cup of grated Parmesan cheese
- 1-1/2 cups of bread flour
- 1 teaspoon of active dry yeast
- 1 cloves garlic, minced
- 1/2 teaspoon of sugar
- 1/2 teaspoon of salt

Direction:

Making the Soup:
1. Place the celery, tomatoes, carrots, onion, broth, and Italian seasoning in a 5-quart slow cooker.
2. Cover and cook for about 7 hours on low.
3. Use an immersion blender to process the soup until smooth.
4. Melt the butter in a saucepan over low-eat just before serving, for about 30 to 45 minutes, stirring constantly.
5. Slowly add the half & half, whisking constantly.
6. Cook mixture until thoroughly smooth and combined.
7. Remove from the heat. Add in the Parmesan cheese, then stir until melted.

8. Add the mixture into the slow cooker. Stir well and cover the slow cooker, then continue cooking for additional 30 minutes.

Making the bread bowls:

9. In a bread machine pan, place the ingredients. Select the dough setting.
10. Turn the dough out on a floured surface when the cycle is complete.
11. Shape the pieces into a ball and place on greased baking sheet.
12. Cover and let it rise until doubled in a warm place for about 30 to 45 minutes.
13. Bake until the bread turns golden brown, for about 18 to 23 minutes, at 400 degrees f.
14. Allow cooling.
15. Serve and enjoy.

Meatballs In A Whole Wheat Bun

Cook Time:
0 minute

Prep Time:
30 minutes

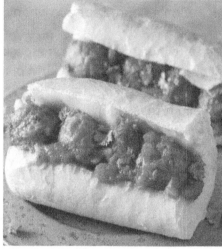

Serving Size
1

Calories per serving:
323kcal

Carbs per serving:
35g

These Meatball Rolls are the perfect Game Day finger good packed with ingredients like balsamic vinegar, oregano, garlic, fresh cremini mushrooms, rosemary, and tomato sauce with mozzarella cheese.

Per Serving:

Fat: 11g | Saturated fat: 3g
Protein: 20g | Fiber: 4g |
Sodium: 600mg | Sugar: 0g

Tip:

You can sprinkle with fresh oregano if you want. Then replace the tops of buns.

Ingredients:

- Nonstick cooking spray
- 1/4 teaspoon of dried rosemary, crushed
- 1/4 teaspoon of dried oregano, crushed
- 3 ounces of refrigerated Italian-style cooked turkey meatballs, halved if desired
- 2 whole wheat frankfurter buns, split
- 1-1/2 cups of thinly sliced fresh cremini mushrooms
- 1/4 cup of chopped onion (1 medium)
- 1 clove garlic, minced
- 1 8 ounces can of no-salt-added tomato sauce
- 1 tablespoon of balsamic vinegar
- 1/8 cup of finely shredded reduced-fat mozzarella cheese
- Snipped fresh oregano (optional)

Direction:

1) Preheat broiler. Use cooking spray to coat a large nonstick skillet.
2) Heat skillet over medium heat and add onions, mushrooms, and garlic, until tender, for about 5 to 10 minutes, stirring occasionally. Stir in balsamic vinegar, tomato sauce, dried oregano, and rosemary. Bring to boiling and reduce heat.
3) Simmer covered for about 2 minutes. Stir in meatballs.
4) Simmer for about 5 minutes, covered until meatballs are heated through.
5) Meanwhile, open buns so they lay flat, then place them on a baking sheet.
6) Broil until lightly toasted, for about 4-inches from the heat.
7) Remove tops of buns from baking sheet and divide meatball mixture among buns' bottoms - sprinkle with cheese.
8) Broil until cheese is melted.
9) Replace tops of buns.
10) Serve, and enjoy.

A Bowl Of Greek Yogurt With Mixed Nuts And Berries

Cook Time:
0 minute

Prep Time:
5 minutes

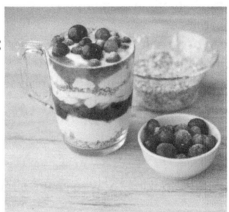

Serving Size
1

Calories per serving:
350kcal

Carbs per serving:
42g

This is a fast and easy lunch that is diabetic friendly. In this recipe, you can use a blend of mixed berries, but fresh berries would be an excellent choice. I hope you enjoy it.

Per Serving:

Fat: 7g | Saturated fat: 0.8g Protein: 29g | Fiber: 6g | Sodium: 120mg | Calcium: 30% DV | Potassium: 200mg | Sugar: 0g

Tip:

This recipe works with just any fruit if you don't have berries on hand.

Ingredients:

- 1 cup of Greek yogurt (plain – I used nonfat, but other varieties will work as well)
- 1/4 cup of oats, granola, or other whole-grain cereal
- 1 cup of mixed berries (thawed if from frozen)
- Whole almonds (about 10 almonds)

Direction:

1. Put all the ingredients together in a variety of ways. It will look great layered in a glass cup or bowl.
2. Use a creamier vanilla yogurt or layer in a bit of maple syrup on top of the yogurt.
3. Toast the nut for maximum flavor and crunch.
4. Serve and enjoy.

Bean And Beef Taco Bowl

Cook Time:
15 minutes

Prep Time:
15 minutes

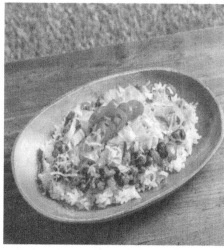

Serving Size
1

Calories per serving:
610kcal

Carbs per serving:
63g

Bean and Beef Taco Bowl are so easy to make at home! They are loaded with seasoned beef taco meat with black beans, layered on rice, and all the taco toppings you want.

Per Serving:

Fat: 22g | **Saturated fat:** 10g
Protein: 42g | **Fiber:** 6g |
Sodium: 870mg | **Potassium:**
0mg | **Sugar:** 5g

Tip:

You can use any leftovers as a filling in quesadillas or burritos.

Ingredients:

- 1/2 tablespoon of canola oil
- 1/2 pound of extra lean ground beef
- 1/2 onion, finely chopped
- 1/2 small red pepper, finely chopped
- 1/2 cup of shredded Monterey Jack cheese
- 1/2 cup of green onions, finely sliced
- 1/3 cup of sour cream
- 1/2 tablespoon of taco seasoning
- 1/2 cup of white rice, cooked according to the package instruction
- 1/2 cup of shredded romaine lettuce
- 1 cup of black beans (canned), rinsed and drained

Direction:

1) In a large skillet, heat oil and set over medium-high heat.
2) Cook onion, beef, and taco seasoning for about 5 to 8 minutes, until meat starts to brown.
3) Stir in 1/4 cup of water.
4) Reduce heat to medium-low.
5) Go ahead with cooking until beef is cooked through, and most of the liquid is evaporated.
6) Top rice with lettuce, beef mixture, black beans, red pepper, salsa, cheese, and green onions.
7) Serve with a dollop of sour cream, if you want.
8) Enjoy.

Pepper And Cottage Cheese Salad Bowl

Cook Time:
0 minute

Prep Time:
10 minutes

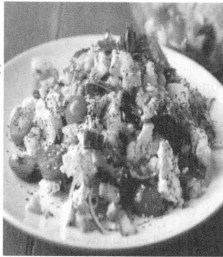

Serving Size
1
**Calories
per serving:**
369kcal
**Carbs
per serving:**
25.4g

Cottage cheese and fresh pepper, french beans, lemon, and hard-boiled eggs make this salad great for lunch! It's light refreshing.Also, it can be adapted in an infinite number of ways.

Per Serving:

Fat: 12.9g | Saturated fat: 4.7g
Protein: 37.3g | Fiber: 7.6g |
Sodium: 738mg | Calcium:
206mg | Potassium: 658mg |
Sugar: 1.2g

Tip:

Before serving, drizzle with oil and season with more pepper and salt.

Ingredients:

- 150grams of cottage cheese
- 2 hard-boiled eggs (yolks discarded)
- Dash of olive oil
- Juice of a lemon
- 30grams of French beans stemmed
- 1 roasted bell pepper with its its juice
- Fresh pepper
- Sea salt

Direction:

1. Preheat oven to 220 degrees c.
2. Roast the peppers until black. Remove from oven and place on a plate, then cover with cling film.
3. In the meantime, boil French beans for about 3 minutes.
4. Remove from hot water and set it aside to cool.
5. Peel the pepper, remove all seeds and tear with hand into strips.
6. Mix the peppers, beans, lemon juice, eggs, olive oil, and seasoning in a bowl.
7. Place on a plate. Arrange cottage cheese on top.
8. Serve and enjoy.

Avocado And Egg On Whole Wheat Toast With Chili Oil

Cook Time:
0 minute

Prep Time:
10 minutes

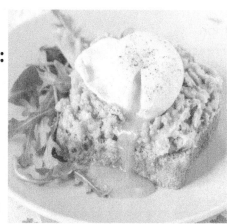

Serving Size
1

Calories per serving:
301kcal

Carbs per serving:
15.2g

If you can try this recipe once, you will agree that topping avocado toast with an egg is a near-perfect lunch.
This recipe is very filling, and you'll want to add it to your favorite lunch.

Per Serving:

Fat: 22.3g | **Saturated fat:** 4.7g
Protein: 14.1g | **Fiber:** 8.1g |
Sodium: 1167mg | **Calcium:**
72mg | **Potassium:** 975mg |
Sugar: 3.1g

Tip:

You can top with a light drizzle of chili oil just before serving, and add some additional salt if needed. 'Flaky sea salt' would be great!

Ingredients:

- 1/4 avocado
- 1 slice whole-wheat bread, toasted
- 1 large egg, fried
- Chili oil, for drizzling
- 1 teaspoon of Sriracha
- 1/4 teaspoon of ground pepper
- 1/8 teaspoon of garlic powder
- 1 tablespoon of scallion, sliced

Direction:

1) Combine pepper, avocado, and garlic powder in a small bowl.
2) Gently mash together.
3) Top the toast with the avocado mixture, fried egg, and lastly, with a light drizzling of chili oil.
4) Serve and enjoy.

Chicken Nuggets

Cook Time:

25 minutes

Prep Time:

15 minutes

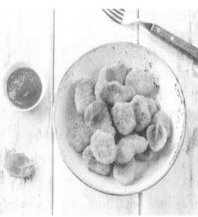

Serving Size

1

Calories per serving:

311kcal

Carbs per serving:

3.1g

Chicken Nuggets are a healthy homemade recipe that is so good for the body. These nuggets require just 6 ingredients to make, and it's super delicious. You may even find yourself craving this healthy version more than you ever craved those fast-food counterparts, and you can enjoy them guilt-free.

Per Serving:

Fat: 24g | **Saturated fat:** 1.5g
Protein: 24g | **Fiber:** 1.6g |
Sodium: 290.8mg | **Calcium:**
31mg | **Potassium:** 3.2mg |
Sugar: 0.5g

Tip:

This dish is best enjoyed immediately and the leftovers can be stored in an airtight container in the refrigerator for up to 3 to 4 days.

Ingredients:

- 1 chicken breasts, (boneless and skinless)
- 1 tablespoon of extra virgin olive oil
- 0.25 teaspoon of salt
- 0.25 cup of almond flour
- 0.5 tablespoon of Italian seasoning
- 0.25 teaspoon of pepper

Direction:

1. Preheat oven to 400 degrees F.
2. Prepare a large baking-sheet using a parchment paper.
3. Stir together the Italian seasoning, almond flour, pepper, and salt in a bowl.
4. Trim any fat off the chicken breast; discard.
5. Then cut into 1-inch thick pieces.
6. Use extra virgin olive oil to spray the chicken.
7. Place each piece into the bowl of flour.
8. Toss until coated, then transfer the chicken into your prepared baking sheet.
9. Bake for about 20 minutes and turn on the broiler.
10. Place the chicken nuggets under the broiler for about 3 to 4 minutes, to make the outside crispy.
11. Serve and enjoy.

Scalloped Potatoes

Cook Time:
0 minute

Prep Time:
50 minutes

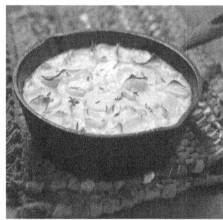

Serving Size
1
Calories per serving:
160kcal
Carbs per serving:
29g

In this dish, thinly sliced onions and potatoes are layered in an easy homemade cream sauce and baked until golden, tender, and bubbly.

Per Serving:

Fat: 2.5g | **Saturated fat:** 1.5g
Protein: 6g | **Fiber:** 2g | **Sodium:** 120mg | **Potassium:** 550mg | **Sugar:** 5g

Tip:

An important step for this recipe is that it needs to be rested. While resting the plate will set.

Ingredients:

- 1 Nonstick cooking spray
- 1 medium yellow onion
- 1/4 teaspoon of black pepper
- 1 cup of fat-free half-and-half
- 1/4 teaspoon of salt (optional)
- 6 medium russet potatoes
- 1/2 cup of cheddar cheese (reduced-fat, shredded sharp, divided)

Direction:

1) Preheat oven to 400 degrees F.
2) Peel the potatoes. Slice into thin rounds.
3) Use cooking spray to coat a large nonstick skillet.
4) Then saute potatoes and onions over medium-high heat until the onions turn clear.
5) Use cooking spray to spray a pie pan and place a thick layer of the potatoes and onion in the bottom of the pan.
6) Add pepper and salt to half-and-half.
7) Pour half cup of the half-and-half over the potatoes.
8) Sprinkle 1/4 cup of the cheese on top, and add the potatoes left, then pour a half cup of half-and-half over the potatoes.
9) Top with the cheese left and bake until potatoes are soft, for about 40 minutes.
10) Serve and enjoy.

Spring Onion And Turkey Wraps

Cook Time:
0 minute

Prep Time:
5 minutes

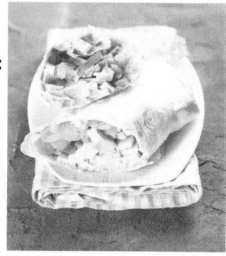

Serving Size
1
Calories per serving:
267kcal
Carbs per serving:
25g

Get yourself a low-fat treat with these super easy and quick sandwich tortillas. This recipe is an excellent way of using up the leftovers turkey. You can apply the dressing to the wrap first to get it distributed evenly; it's your choice!

Per Serving:

Fat: 9g | Saturated fat: 2g
Protein: 24g | Fiber: 2g | Sugar: 3g

Tip:

You can use leftover turkey for this recipe.

Ingredients:

- 2 tablespoons of reduced-fat mayonnaise
- 2 tablespoons of pesto
- 12cm chunk cucumber, shredded
- 4 flour tortillas
- 4 curly lettuce leaves
- 250grams of cooked turkey, shredded
- 6 spring onions, shredded

Direction:

1. Mix the pesto and mayonnaise together.
2. Divide the lettuce leaves, spring onions, turkey, and cucumber between the tortillas.
3. Drizzle over the pesto dressing.
4. Roll up.
5. Eat and enjoy it.

Chickpea Curry

Cook Time:

15 minutes

Prep Time:

5 minutes

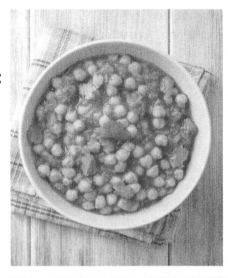

Serving Size

1

Calories per serving:

278.2kcal

Carbs per serving:

30.3g

This recipe is made with convenient canned beans and is an authentic chickpea curry that you can make within 15 minutes. You can stir in some roasted cauliflower florets if you want an additional vegetable. It's a lunch recipe that goes with basmati rice or warm rice. You would love it!

Per Serving:

Fat: 15.5g | Saturated fat: 1.2g
Protein: 5.8g | Fiber: 6.3g |
Sodium: 354.2mg | Calcium:
65.3mg | Potassium: 355.7mg |
Sugar: 3.1g

Tip:

Before serving, you can top with cilantro, if you feel like.

Ingredients:

- 1 medium serrano pepper, cut into thirds
- 2 teaspoons of ground coriander
- 2 teaspoons of ground cumin
- 1/2 teaspoon of ground turmeric
- 2-1/4 cups of no-salt-added canned diced tomatoes with their juice (from a 28-ounce can)
- 3/4 teaspoon of kosher salt
- 4 large cloves garlic
- 1 2-inch piece of fresh ginger, peeled and coarsely chopped
- 1 medium yellow onion, chopped (1-inch)
- 6 tablespoons of canola oil or grapeseed oil
- 2 15-ounce cans of chickpeas, rinsed
- 2 teaspoons of garam masala
- 1 Fresh cilantro for garnish

Direction:

1) In a food processor, pulse serrano, ginger, and garlic until minced. Scrape down the sides and pulse again.
2) Add onion; pulse until finely chopped (not watery)
3) In a large saucepan, heat oil over medium-high heat.
4) Add the onion mixture and cook. Stir occasionally, for about 5 minutes, until softened. Add cumin, coriander, and turmeric and cook, stirring, for about 2 minutes.
5) Pulse the tomatoes in the food processor until finely chopped.
6) Add the pan along with the salt.
7) Reduce heat to maintain a simmer, then cook, occasionally stirring for about 4 minutes.
8) Add garam masala and chickpeas, reduce heat to a gentle simmer. Then cover and cook. Stirring occasionally, for another 5 minutes. Serve topped with cilantro if you want.
9) Enjoy.

Dinner Recipes

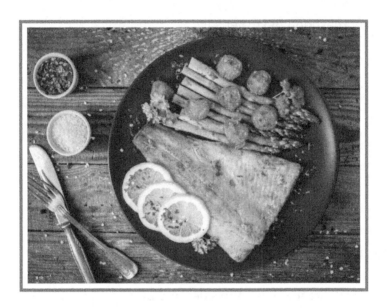

Salmon And Spinach With Avocado

0 minute

Prep Time:
10 minutes

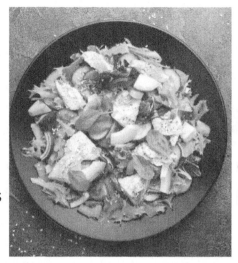

1

**Calories
per serving:**
301kcal

**Carbs
per serving:**
15.2g

This recipe is packed with nutrients that will keep you full longer and make you healthier. I highly recommend this recipe if you would like to lose weight, and it's best for diabetic people. So you need to increase your intake of vegetables and fruits, making this an ideal meal excellent to-go!

Per Serving:

Fat: 22.3g | **Saturated fat:** 4.7g
Protein: 14.1g | **Fiber:** 8.1g |
Sodium: 1167mg | **Calcium:**
72mg | **Potassium:** 975mg |
Sugar: 3.1g

Tip:

You can top with a light drizzle of chili oil just before serving, and add some additional salt if needed. Flaky sea salt would be great!

Ingredients:

- 1 cup of baby spinach
- 2 ounces of smoked salmon
- 1/2 Haas avocado
- 1/2 cucumber, thinly sliced
- 1 medium sized tomatoes

For the dressing:
- 1/2 lime juice
- 0.25 cup of extra virgin olive oil
- Himalayan sea salt
- fresh ground pepper

Direction:

For the dressing:
1. Squeeze the juice of one lime inside a small bowl.
2. Add the extra virgin olive oil.
3. Whisk together until thoroughly combined.

4. Season with fresh ground pepper and Himalayan sea salt.

Add the salad:
5. Add the spinach into a salad bowl.
6. Slice the cucumber, avocado, and tomatoes; then add them into the spinach.
7. Slice the salmon and add them into the bowl also.
8. Drizzle the dressing over the salad.
9. Serve and enjoy.

Salmon With Quinoa And Vegetable Stir-Fry

Cook Time:
20 minute

Prep Time:
15 minutes

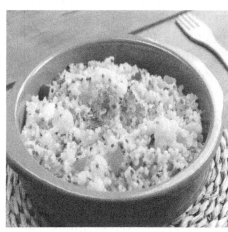

Serving Size
1

Calories per serving:
447kcal

Carbs per serving:
40g

Quinoa is similar to rice except that it has a crunchier texture, fluffier and nuttier. So it can be done in the rice cooker! It would be best if you cook more quinoa because it's so healthy and hearty. You need to use the Chinese chives in this dish; it gives the dish a garlicky flavor! Having it with salmon is mouthwatering.

Per Serving:

Fat: 9.4g | Saturated fat: 1.8g
Protein: 44.8g | Fiber: 0g |
Sodium: 209mg | Sugar: 15.5g

Tip:

You can add some feta to the salad if you like, or some fresh baby spinach leaves.

Ingredients:

- 0.5 cup of quinoa (200g)
- 1 tablespoon of vegetable oil
- 1 cloves garlic (minced)
- 4 ounces of cooked salmon (flaked) (225g)
- 1 tablespoon of soy sauce
- Salt and pepper to taste
- 0.5 small carrot (peeled and finely cubed)
- 0.5 cup of corn kernel (150g)
- 1 ounce of Chinese chives (thinly sliced) (60g)

Direction:

1) Rinse quinoa until water runs clear. In a medium-sized pan, drain and place the quinoa, then add 2 cups of water. Place it on a stove, and bring water to boil.
2) Decrease heat and let the quinoa simmer for about 15 minutes, until water is absorbed.
3) Turn off the heat and use a fork to fluff the quinoa to allow it to cool completely.
4) Heat the veggie oil in a large non-stick fry-pan.
5) Fry garlic for about 1 minute. Add corn and carrots, then fry for 2 to 3 minutes.
6) Add chives and salmon. Then cook for another minute.
7) Then add your cooked quinoa. Stir to combine all the ingredients.
8) Add salt, soy sauce, and pepper.
9) Stir to get everything well combined and cook until quinoa is fluffy and dry. This will take about 5 minutes.
10) Remove and serve immediately.
11) Enjoy.

Chicken And Vegetable Stir-Fry

Cook Time:
10 minutes

Prep Time:
10 minutes

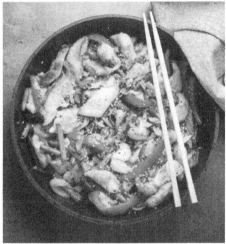

Serving Size
1

Calories per serving:
180kcal

Carbs per serving:
9g

This Chicken and Vegetable Stir-fry is a perfect way to make a diabetes-friendly, healthy, and low-carb meal from whatever you might have in your pantry or fridge. You need to give this recipe a try today!

Per Serving:

Fat: 8g | **Saturated fat:** 1.5g
Protein: 18g | **Fiber:** 2g |
Sodium: 380mg | **Potassium:**
530mg | **Sugar:** 3g

Tip:

You can let it cool then store in an airtight container in the refrigerator for up to 7 days.

Ingredients:

- 1 clove of garlic (grated or minced)
- 1 tablespoon of olive oil
- 1/2 teaspoon of ground black pepper
- 1-1/2 cup of cooked chicken (shredded)
- 1 cup of low sodium chicken broth
- 2 teaspoons of corn starch
- 1 14-ounces bag of frozen stir-fry vegetables
- 2 tablespoons of lower-sodium soy sauce

Direction:

1. Add olive oil into a non-stick skillet over high heat.
2. Add the frozen vegetables, then saute for about 5 minutes.
3. While the vegetables are sauteing, whisk the soy sauce, broth, garlic, corn starch, and black pepper in a bowl until well combined.
4. Add the sauce and chicken into the pan.
5. Saute until chicken is heated through and sauce is thickened, for about 5 minutes.
6. Serve and enjoy.

Spicy Chicken And Quinoa

Cook Time:
25 minute

Prep Time:
15 minutes

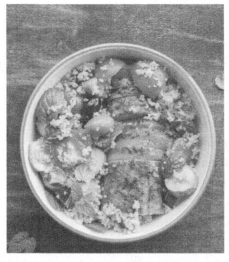

Serving Size
1
Calories per serving:
673kcal
Carbs per serving:
73.8g

This is a great dinner salad that will take about 20 minutes to cook. You can omit the chili if you don't like spicy foods. Instead of quinoa, you can use couscous, freekeh, or even brown rice. You can also have the option to add some feta to the salad or some fresh baby spinach leaves. I hope you enjoy eating it.

Per Serving:

Fat: 26.7g | **Saturated fat:** 4.4g
Protein: 37.9g | **Fiber:** 8.9g |
Sodium: 1411mg | **Calcium:**
97mg | **Potassium:** 1250mg |
Sugar: 4g

Tip:

You can use Chinese chives to give the dish a garlicky flavor.

Ingredients:

- 1/2 large chicken breast
- 0.25 cup of quinoa, dried
- 1/2 teaspoon of olive oil
- 4 cherry tomatoes, halved
- 1/2 small cumber, diced
- 70grams of green beans, halved
- 1/2 spring onion, sliced
- 1/2 large lemon juiced
- 1/2 large orange, juiced
- 1/2 tablespoon of honey
- 1/2 cup of water
- 1/4 teaspoon of chili powder or flakes
- 1/2 teaspoon of paprika
- 1/2 teaspoon of smoked paprika
- 1/2 teaspoon of season all
- 1/2 teaspoon of cracked pepper

Direction:

1) In a pot, place your water and quinoa, bring to boil, and simmer for about 10 min.
2) Take off the heat and use your fork to fluff. Place into a large mixing bowl. Add tomatoes, cucumber, and spring onion into the mixing bowl, and mix. Heat 1 pot of water to blanch the beans. Simmer for 2 mins, then place into cold water, for about a minute, and drain on a paper towel, then place into the mixing bowl.
3) Place your paprika, chili, pepper into a bowl, and mix.
4) Cut the chicken into strips. Place them into your bowl. Mix with seasoning until the chicken has been coated.
5) Drizzle over the olive oil and mix.
6) Heat a non-stick griddle pan. Then cook the chicken.
7) Mix your fresh lemon and orange juice in a small bowl, heat the honey in the microwave for about 20 seconds, and mix with the juices. Mix in with the quinoa and salad mixture.
8) Place into the serving plate with the chicken on top. Enjoy.

Spinach, Apple, And Chicken Salad

Cook Time:
0 minute

Prep Time:
20 minutes

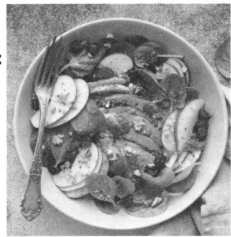

Serving Size
1

Calories per serving:
348.7kcal

Carbs per serving:
26.1g

Swap out store-bought for this tangy poppy seed dressing and homemade buttermilk to make this healthy salad recipe to the next level. Make your crunchy cheese crisps in a snap, using phyllo dough, for a delicious accompaniment to this dinner salad.
I hope you enjoy it!

Per Serving:

Fat: 16.7g | Saturated fat: 3.6g
Protein: 23.1g | Fiber: 3.3g |
Sodium: 566.7mg | Calcium:
189.7mg | Potassium: 249mg |
Sugar: 14.1g

Tip:

If you want to make this dish ahead, refrigerate dressing for up to 2 days.

Ingredients:

- 3 eaches 9-by-14-inch of phyllo pastry sheets, thawed
- 3 tablespoons of buttermilk
- 2 tablespoons of honey
- 1 tablespoon of cider vinegar
- 1 teaspoon of poppy seeds
- 1/2 teaspoon of Dijon mustard
- 1/2 teaspoon of kosher salt
- 5 cups of baby spinach
- 4 teaspoons of extra-virgin olive oil plus 2 tablespoons, divided
- 1 large egg white, beaten
- 1/3 cup of freshly grated Parmigiano-Reggiano cheese
- 1 tablespoon of fresh thyme leaves
- 1-1/2 cups of shredded cooked chicken breast
- 1 medium Gala apple, sliced

Direction:

1. Preheat oven to 350 degrees f.
2. Use parchment paper to line a baking sheet.
3. Place 1 sheet of phyllo on the prepared baking sheet, and use 2 teaspoons of oil to brush.
4. Top with the second sheet of phyllo, but gently pressing to adhere; use 2 teaspoons of oil to brush again.
5. Place the third sheet on top, and finally, brush with egg white.
6. Sprinkle with thyme and cheese.
7. Cut the phyllo stack into approx. 2-inch squares using a sharp knife. Bake for about 8 minutes, until golden brown, and let it cool for about 3 minutes.
8. Meanwhile, whisk the buttermilk, the remaining 2 tablespoons of oil, honey, poppy seeds, vinegar, salt, and mustard in a medium bowl. Add the chicken, spinach, and apple into the bowl, then toss to coat.
9. Serve with the phyllo crisps. Enjoy.

Leafy Green Salmon Salad With Sesame Seeds

Cook Time:
20 minute

Prep Time:
10 minutes

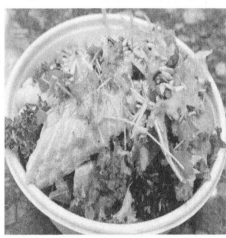

Serving Size
1

Calories per serving:
433kcal

Carbs per serving:
30.5g

This Leafy Green Salmon Salad with Sesame Seeds is healthy, light, and full of flavor. Salmon is incredibly tasty when paired with leafy greens, avocado, a refreshing vinaigrette, and no-too-sweet marinade.
Here you have it - enjoy!

Per Serving:

Fat: 34.9g | **Saturated fat:** 6.4g
Protein: 5.8g | **Fiber:** 9.5g |
Sodium: 726mg | **Calcium:**
100mg | **Potassium:** 1043mg |
Sugar: 10.5g

Tip:

You can squeeze a bit of extra lemon juice on top of the salad just before serving.

Ingredients:

- 1 piece salmon
- 1/2 avocado
- Cucumber to taste
- Salad greens (you can use a spring mix + butter leaf lettuce)
- Spring onions to taste
- **Marinade:**
- 1/2 tablespoon of soy sauce
- 1 tablespoon of hoisin sauce
- 1/2 teaspoon of ground ginger
- 1 clove garlic minced
- **Dressing:**
- 1/2 teaspoon of rice vinegar
- 0.75 teaspoon of lemon juice
- 1/2 pinch of ground ginger
- 1 tablespoon of sesame oil
- 1/2 clove garlic minced
- 1/2 teaspoon of toasted sesame seeds
- Salt & pepper to taste

Direction:

1) Marinate the salmon before cooking for about 30 to 60 minutes.
   Making the marinade:
2) Add all the marinade ingredients together in a Ziploc bag. Add the fish, then place it in the fridge.
3) Preheat oven to 375 degrees f when the salmon is almost finished marinating.
4) Meanwhile, make the dressing by adding all the dressing ingredients except the sesame seeds.
5) In a small pan on high heat, place the sesame seeds to toast them.
6) Watch them carefully, then shake the pan so as to spread them around for about 5 minutes (note that they can burn fast).

7) Remove from heat when they turn a light brown color.
8) Let them cool. Then add them into the dressing.
9) Add to a foil-lined baking sheet once salmon is finished marinating, and bake for about 10 to 15 minutes, or until cooked through.
10) Prepare the salad by slicing the cucumber, avocado, and spring onions while salmon is cooking. Then toss them with the salad greens and dressing.
11) Top salad with the cooked salmon.
12) Serve and enjoy.

Rosemary Pork Chops With Roasted Cauliflower

Cook Time:

20 minutes

Prep Time:

10 minutes

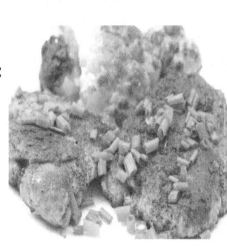

Serving Size

1

Calories per serving:

296.5kcal

Carbs per serving:

11g

This quick one-skillet vegetable and pork main dish recipe make an excellent weeknight dinner. Look for pre-cut cauliflower florets in any grocery store around you to cut down on prep time, and your dinner will be ready on the table in just 30 minutes.

Per Serving:

Fat: 13.8g | Saturated fat: 3.4g
Protein: 31.9g | Fiber: 4.3g |
Sodium: 389.2mg | Calcium:
63.8mg | Potassium: 963.4mg |
Sugar: 4.2g

Tip:

Sprinkle the vegetable mixture with parsley/chives and basil.

Ingredients:

- 2 raw chop with refuse, 113 grams; (blank) 4 ounces of pork rib chops, cut 3/4 inch thick (8 ounces total)
- 2 teaspoons chopped of fresh thyme or 1/2 teaspoon dried, crushed
- 1/4 teaspoon of salt, divided
- 1/4 teaspoon of freshly ground pepper, divided
- 3 cups of cauliflower florets
- 1 small onion, cut into wedges
- 1 tablespoon of olive oil
- 1 leaf chopped of fresh basil, Italian parsley, and/or chives.

Direction:

1. Trim fat from meat. Stir together 1/8 teaspoon of salt, thyme, and 1/8 teaspoon of pepper in a small bowl.
2. Sprinkle evenly on both sides of each chop and rub in using your fingers. Set the chops aside.
3. Use cooking spray to coat a very large unheated nonstick.
4. Preheat over medium-high heat and add onion with cauliflower; sprinkle the remaining 1/8 teaspoon of pepper and salt.
5. Cook and stir until almost tender, for about 5 minutes.
6. Remove skillet from heat and push onion and cauliflower to the edge of the skillet. Add oil to the skillet and in a single layer, arrange the seasoned chops in the skillet.
7. Return the skillet to the heat and cook over medium heat until the pork chops are done, and vegetables are tender, for about 10 minutes, turning the chops to brown evenly.
8. Add oil to the skillet and in a single layer, arrange seasoned chops in skillet.
9. Cook until pork chops are done, and vegetables are tender, for about 10 minutes, stirring vegetables often and turning chops to brown evenly.
10. Transfer the vegetables and chops mixture into the dinner plates.
11. Serve and enjoy.

Grilled Chicken With Roasted Cauliflower And Quinoa

Cook Time:
30 minutes

Prep Time:
10 minutes

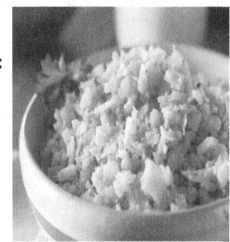

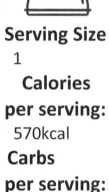

Serving Size
1
Calories per serving:
570kcal
Carbs per serving:
57.7g

A typically European approach to cooking chicken is roasting it with a lemon. To get this ready to eat, all you need to do is add a delicious quinoa medley, carrot, cauliflower, garlic, onion, grated zucchini, mint & a hit of lemon juice, and then you've got a deliciously healthy dinner on your hands. I hope you enjoy it!

Per Serving:

Fat: 14.5g | Saturated fat: 0g
Protein: 48.3g | Fiber: 0g |
Sodium: 0mg | Calcium: 0mg |
Potassium: 0mg | Sugar: 0g

Tip:

Enjoy this salad with Quinoa, lemon and mint.

Ingredients:

- Onion
- Cauliflower
- Carrots
- Garlic
- 2 extra virgin olive oil
- Salt and pepper
- 1 lemon slices
- chicken breasts
- 450milliltre of water
- Quinoa
- Zucchini
- Mint leaves

Direction:

1) Heat the oven to 200 degrees C, fan-forced.
2) Use baking paper to line 2 oven trays, then cut the onion into wedges, and cauliflower into small florets.
3) Peel the carrots, and cut into 1cm chunks.
4) Finely chop the garlic.
5) Then place cauliflower, carrot, onions, and garlic on a lined tray.
6) Add 2 tablespoons of extra virgin olive oil and season with pepper and salt. Toss to combine.
7) Slice half of the lemon and juice the remaining half.
8) Place the chicken breasts on the rest of the lined tray.
9) Season with pepper and salt, then spray with olive oil and place the lemon slices just on top of the chicken.
10) Roast the vegetables and chicken until the chicken is cooked through and vegetables are tender for about 20 minutes.
11) Meanwhile, in a sieve, put the quinoa and then rinse well. Drain it and in a medium saucepan, put the quinoa with 450ml of water, cover, then bring to a simmer.
12) Reduce the heat to low and cook, covered until the quinoa is tender and water is absorbed for about 15 minutes.
13) Turn off the heat and stand, covered, for about 5 minutes.

14) Rest the chicken for about 5 minutes. Coarsely grate the zucchini while the chicken is resting.
15) Chop the mint leaves finely, discarding the stems.
16) Reserve the lemon slices from the chicken and slice the chicken.
17) Put the roasted vegetable, quinoa, 1 tablespoon of lemon juice, zucchini, and mint in a large bowl.
18) Season with pepper and salt, and toss to combine.
19) Serve and enjoy.

Grilled Chicken Chopped Salad

Cook Time:
30 minutes

Prep Time:
5 minutes

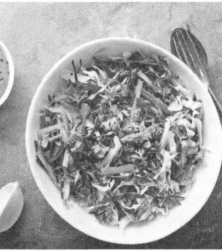

Serving Size
1

Calories per serving:
329kcal

Carbs per serving:
14.7g

Grilled Chicken Chopped Salad utilizes vegetables topped with easy baked chicken with seasonal fruits to create a hearthy, colorful, and protein-packed salad.

Per Serving:

Fat: 16.6g | **Saturated fat:** 3.7g
Protein: 30.6g | **Fiber:** 3.8g |
Sodium: 415.3mg | **Calcium:**
117mg | **Potassium:** 675.8mg |
Sugar: 5.2g

Tip:

Fennel isn't easy to find. So it can be omitted or substituted with celery.

Ingredients:

Baked Chicken:
- 0.33 pound of boneless skinless chicken thighs
- 0.08 teaspoon of garlic powder
- 0.08 teaspoon of onion powder
- Olive oil spray
- 0.08 teaspoon of pepper
- 0.08 teaspoon of salt

Salad:
- 0.5 cups of kale, chopped in bite-sized pieces
- 0.17 small stalk of fennel, sliced thinly (divided)
- 0.04 cup of pomegranate seeds
- 0.17 cucumber, chopped in bite-sized pieces
- 0.17 tomato, diced
- 0.17 cup of Brussels sprouts, chopped into bite-sized slices
- 0.17 cup of purple cabbage, sliced
- 0.17 carrot, cut in ribbons with a mandolin (or sliced thinly)
- 0.17 red onion, sliced thinly
- 0.04 cup of crumbled feta (optional)

Garlic Citrus Vinaigrette:
- 0.08 teaspoon of salt
- 0.08 teaspoon of pepper
- 0.17 garlic cloves, minced
- 0.04 cup of extra virgin olive oil
- 0.25 lemons, juiced (approximately 4 tablespoons of juice)
- 0.17 teaspoon of minced fennel

Direction:
1. Preheat oven to 375 degrees F.
2. Use olive oil to spray a small pan.

3. Spread seasonings on both sides of the chicken thighs.
4. Place in pan and bake until the thickest part of the thigh reads 165 degrees for about 30 minutes.
5. Set it aside and allow it to cool.
6. Prepare the salad ingredients while the chicken is baking.
7. Chop the Brussels sprouts, kale, and cucumber.
8. Slice the put cabbage, red onion, carrot, and fennel thinly, then dice the tomato.
9. In a large bowl, toss the ingredients, then place in the refrigerator until needed.
10. Add all the vinaigrette ingredients in a mason jar, then vigorously shake.
11. Place in the refrigerator until needed.
12. Chop into bite-sized pieces once the chicken has cooled.
13. Place over salad and drizzle on the vinaigrette.
14. Then toss, serve, and enjoy.

Thai Stir-Fry With Pork Strips

Cook Time:
30 minutes

Prep Time:
5 minutes

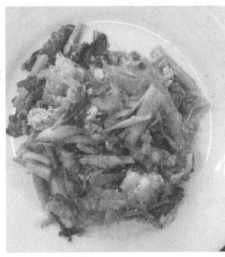

Serving Size
1

Calories per serving:
281.9kcal

Carbs per serving:
23.2g

Thai Stir-Fry With Pork Strips is a 30 minutes dinner recipe you would love. Cardamom, ginger, curry powder are just some of the many spices that lend flavor to the pork.

Per Serving:

Fat: 8.1g | **Saturated fat:** 2.9g
Protein: 26g | **Fiber:** 2.4g |
Sodium: 321.2mg | **Calcium:**
12.5mg | **Potassium:** 482.5mg |
Sugar: 4.3g

Tip:

Choose natural pork rather than enhanced pork to keep the sodium in this dish in check.

Ingredients:

- 2 tablespoons of olive oil
- 1/2 teaspoon of ground cardamom
- 1/2 teaspoon of chili powder
- 1 1/2 pounds of pork loin, cut into bite-size strips
- 2 cups of broccoli florets
- 1 cup of thinly sliced carrots
- 1 cup of cauliflower florets
- 2 tablespoons of white vinegar
- 1 tablespoon of curry powder
- 1 tablespoon of reduced-sodium soy sauce
- 1/2 teaspoon of garlic powder
- 1/2 teaspoon of finely chopped fresh ginger or 1/4 teaspoon of ground ginger
- 1/2 teaspoon of ground black pepper
- 2 cups of hot cooked brown rice

Direction:

1) In a very large skillet, combine soy sauce, oil, garlic powder, pepper, ginger, oil, chili powder, and cardamom.
2) Add half of the pork; stir-fry pork over medium-high heat for about 3 minutes.
3) Remove pork from skillet using a slotted spoon.
4) Repeat with the rest of the pork.
5) Return all of the pork into the skillet.
6) Add carrot, broccoli, vinegar, cauliflower, and curry powder to the pork mixture.
7) Bring to boiling and reduce heat.
8) Cover and simmer until vegetables are crisp-tender, for about 3 to 5 minutes, stirring occasionally.
9) Serve vegetables and pork over brown rice.
10) Enjoy!

Spicy Pork Tacos

Cook Time:
0 minute

Prep Time:
45 minutes

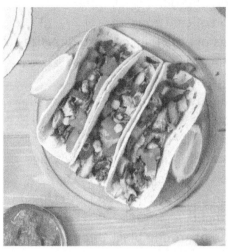

Serving Size
1

Calories per serving:
130kcal

Carbs per serving:
13g

This recipe calls for pork tenderloin. Spicy Pork Tacos you can have with fresh salsa and avocado. The addition of cheese makes me love this recipe so much, and I'm sure you'll enjoy it as well.

Per Serving:

Fat: 5g | Saturated fat: 1.5g
Protein: 16g | Fiber: 8g |
Sodium: 400mg

Tip:

You can also top this tacos with fresh salsa and avocado.

Ingredients:

- 1/2 juiced lime
- 1/2 clove garlic
- 1/2 tablespoons of chili powder
- 1/4 teaspoon of cumin
- 1 tomato
- 1/2 cup of lettuce
- 1/4 cup of cheddar cheese
- 1/4 teaspoon of dried oregano
- 1/4 teaspoon of salt
- 1/4 teaspoon of black pepper
- 1/2 pork tenderloin
- 1 tortilla

Direction:

1. Combine lime juice, garlic, cumin, chili powder, oregano, pepper, and salt in a large bowl.
2. Add pork and coat well.
3. Marinate for about 30 minutes up to 4 hours in the refrigerator.
4. Preheat oven to 375 degrees.
5. In a shallow baking dish, place tenderloins and bake until pork is done for about 30 minutes.
6. Remove pork from the oven and let it rest for about 10 minutes.
7. Cut pork into 1-inch chunks.
8. Serve pork in a warm tortilla topped with tomatoes, lettuce, and cheese.
9. Enjoy.

Chicken And Quinoa One-Pot With Broccoli

Cook Time:

30 minutes

Prep Time:

5 minutes

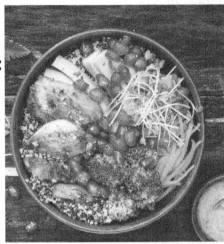

Serving Size

1

Calories per serving:

240.3kcal

Carbs per serving:

21.5g

Roasting lemons mellow their tartness. It also creates a layer of caramelized flavor which pairs well with the savory quinoa and raw broccoli in this healthy chicken dinner salad. This is one of the best delicious meal that is so easy to make.

Per Serving:

Fat: 13.3g | **Saturated fat:** 1.6g **Protein:** 10.8g | **Fiber:** 4g | **Sodium:** 182.3mg | **Calcium:** 70mg | **Potassium:** 292.3mg | **Sugar:** 7.10g

Tip:

You can reduce the lemon if it's too lemony, but I love it that way.

Ingredients:

- 1 (8 ounces) of boneless, skinless chicken breast, trimmed
- 4 tablespoons of extra-virgin olive oil, divided
- 1/8 teaspoon of salt plus 1/4 teaspoon, divided
- 2 small lemons, thinly sliced and seeded
- 1 tablespoon of Dijon mustard
- 2 cups of arugula
- 3/4 cup of chopped walnuts, toasted
- 1/2 cup of dried cranberries
- 1/2 cup of chopped fresh mint
- 1 cup of low-sodium chicken broth
- 1/2 cup of quinoa
- 8 ounces of broccoli with stems (about 1 medium head)
- 1/4 cup of red-wine vinegar

Direction:

1) Preheat oven to 425 degrees F. Place chicken on a side of the rimmed baking sheet, drizzle 1 tablespoon of oil, and then sprinkle the salt. Roast for about 10 minutes, and place lemon slices on the other side of the baking sheet.
2) Roast till a thermometer inserted into the thickest part of the chicken reaches 160 degrees F, and the lemon is browned, turning once, for about 7 to 9 minutes more.
3) Meanwhile, in a small saucepan, bring quinoa & broth to boil.
4) Reduce heat to maintain a simmer, cover, and cook until the liquid is absorbed, for about 15 min. Remove from heat. Let it stand, covered, for about 10-min. Cut broccoli florets from the stems. Trim, peel and slice the stems thinly, and chop the florets into bite-size pieces. Chop half of the lemon slices. Combine mustard, vinegar, the remaining oil, and 1/4 teaspoon of salt in a large bowl.
5) Shred the chicken and add both the chicken, the rest of the lemon slices, broccoli, arugula, quinoa, walnuts, mint, and cranberries into the dressing. Toss, serve, and enjoy.

Chicken And Vegetable Bowl With Cottage Cheese

Cook Time:
30 minute

Prep Time:
5 minutes

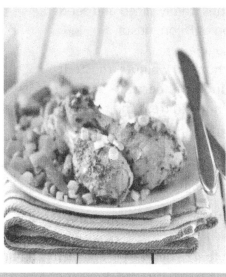

Serving Size
1

Calories per serving:
354kcal

Carbs per serving:
17g

Chicken and Vegetable Bowl With Cottage Cheese is loaded with veggies, tender, and cheese, juicy chicken that can be made within 30 minutes. It's also a one-skillet dinner that is fast, easy and, most of all, delicious!

Per Serving:

Fat: 14g | **Saturated fat:** 4g
Protein: 38g | **Fiber:** 5g |
Sodium: 451mg | **Calcium:**
261mg | **Potassium:** 735mg |
Sugar: 1g

Tip:

It's not necessary you drain the water after cooking the veggies. The water will evaporate.

Ingredients:

- 1 boneless, skinless chicken breasts
- 0.25 bag (16-ounces) vegetable blend
- 0.25 jar (4-ounces) of diced pimientos
- 0.25 cup of shredded cheddar cheese
- 0.5 tablespoon of olive oil
- salt and fresh ground pepper, to taste
- 0.25 cup of water
- 0.13- a cup of part-skim shredded mozzarella cheese
- chopped fresh parsley, for garnish

Direction:

1. Pound chicken lightly, just enough to even it out. Make sure you don't pound it thin.
2. Over medium-high heat, heat the olive oil.
3. Add chicken—season with pepper and salt.
4. Cover and cook until browned, for about 5 minutes on each side.
5. Remove chicken from skillet and set it aside.
6. Add frozen vegetables & water to skillet; bring to a boil.
7. Lower to a simmer. Cover and cook for about 3 minutes.
8. Add chicken back into the skillet.
9. Stir in diced pimientos. Sprinkle cheese over vegetables and chicken.
10. Cover & cook until cheese is melted and chicken is cooked thoroughly over medium heat for about 5 minutes.
11. Remove from heat. Garnish with parsley.
12. Serve and enjoy.

Lentils And Green Salad With Dressing

Cook Time:
0 minute

Prep Time:
20 minutes

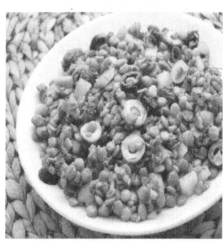

Serving Size
1

Calories per serving:
170kcal

Carbs per serving:
21g

This recipe is a very quick recipe that is ready can be ready in just 20 minutes. It's not necessary to soak dry lentils before cooking. It's perfect that way.

Per Serving:

Fat: 7g | **Saturated fat:** 1g
Protein: 9g | **Fiber:** 8g | **Sodium:** 5mg | **Potassium:** 440mg | **Sugar:** 3g

Tip:

Refrigerate until you're ready to serve.

Ingredients:

- 1/2 cup of lentils (sorted & rinsed)
- 1/5 cup of water
- 1 clove garlic (sliced in half)
- 1 green onion (sliced)
- 2 tablespoons of olive oil
- 1/4 teaspoon of parsley(dried)
- 1/4 teaspoon of black pepper
- 1/4 cup of green pepper (diced)
- 1/2 cup of grape tomatoes (halved)
- 1 Juice of 1 lemon

Direction:

1) Combine water, lentils, and garlic in a pot over medium heat.
2) Simmer until the lentils are tender for about 15 minutes.
3) Drain lentils and run under cold water.
4) Discard the garlic.
5) Whisk together the dressing ingredients while the lentils are cooking.
6) In a salad bowl, add lentils, green pepper, green onion, and tomatoes.
7) Drizzle dressing over the lentils then mix to combine.
8) Refrigerate until serving.
9) Serve and enjoy.

Salmon And Pepper With Green Salad

Cook Time:
0 minute

Prep Time:
5 minutes

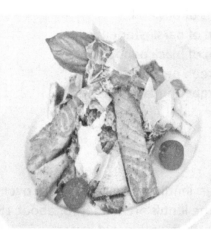

Serving Size
1

Calories per serving:
531kcal

Carbs per serving:
20g

I recommend cutting your chopped romaine very fine or buying it already chopped like that in this recipe. Then, toss your lettuce in the amount of dressing you want along with the toppings, then everything will be perfectly mixed together. Enjoy!

Per Serving:

Tip:

Fat: 30g | **Saturated fat:** 6g
Protein: 48g | **Fiber:** 11g |
Sugar: 4.5g

Top your green salad with avocado and cooked salmon.

Ingredients:

- 5 ounces of finely chopped romaine leaves (about 3-4 cups)
- 2 tablespoons of Marie's Smoked Black Pepper Caesar Dressing
- 1/2 small avocado chopped
- 6 ounces of salmon filet (cook as desired)
- 1/2 cup of broccoli florets chopped
- 1/4 cup of chopped red bell pepper
- 1/4 cup of Parmesan flakes

Direction:

1. Gently toss the chopped romaine in a large bowl with Marie's Smoked Black Pepper Caesar Dressing, Parmesan, broccoli, and red bell pepper.
2. Transfer the salad to a serving bowl.
3. Top with the cooked salmon and avocado.
4. Serve and enjoy.

Lemon And Herb Chicken With Brown Rice

Cook Time:
1 hr 35 min

Prep Time:
50 minutes

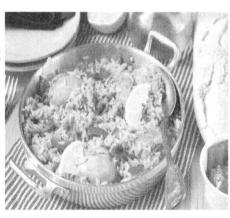

Serving Size
1

Calories per serving:
273.7kcal

Carbs per serving:
29.4g

This easy dish has a beautiful golden color and a wonderful fragrance. You need to add that saffron in the cupboard; just a little will enhance the dish's aroma and flavor. As for me, I will make this recipe 10 times!

Per Serving:

Fat: 9.7g | **Saturated fat:** 2.2g
Protein: 17g | **Fiber:** 3.3g |
Sodium: 194.5mg | **Calcium:**
39.1mg | **Potassium:** 307.5mg |
Sugar: 2.7g

Tip:

You can bake the full recipe in a 9x13 inch baking pan instead of freezing half - in step 13.

Ingredients:

- 2 tablespoons of olive oil, divided
- 1 pinch of Generous pinch of saffron
- 3 cups of shredded cabbage (about 1/2 small head)
- 4 cups of cooked brown rice, preferably basmati or jasmine
- 1/4 cup of lemon juice
- 8 eaches boneless, skinless chicken thighs, trimmed
- 2 large onions, thinly sliced
- 1/2 teaspoon of salt, divided
- 3 cloves garlic, minced
- 2 teaspoons of ground turmeric
- 1 teaspoon of paprika
- 2 tablespoons of chopped fresh Italian parsley
- 1 lemon, sliced

Direction:

1) Preheat oven to 375 degrees F.
2) Coat two 8-inch-square baking dishes.
3) In a large nonstick skillet, heat 1 tablespoon of oil over medium-high heat.
4) Add 4 chicken thighs. Then cook, turning once, for about 4 minutes, until both sides are lightly browned.
5) Transfer the chicken into a plate, and set it aside.
6) Repeat with the rest of the chicken thighs and pour off all, but about 1 tablespoon of fat from the pan.
7) Add the onions and the remaining 1 tablespoon of oil to the pan. Sprinkle with 1/4 teaspoon of salt. Cook, stirring, for about 15 minutes, until golden and soft. Stir in garlic, paprika, turmeric, and saffron, if using; stir and cook for 2 minutes. Transfer the onions into a plate and set it aside.
8) Return the pan to medium-high heat, then add cabbage. Cook, stirring for about 3 minutes until wilted.

9) Stir in lemon juice, rice, half of the reserved onion, and the rest of the salt.
10) Continue cooking for about 5 minutes, until the rice is well coated and heated through.
11) Divide the rice mixture between the prepared baking dishes; nestle 4 of the reserved chicken thighs in each dish.
12) Top each with half of the cooked onions left. Cover both dishes with foil, and freeze 1 of them for up to 1 month.
13) Bake the remaining casserole for 30 minutes, but covered.
14) Uncover and continue baking until the onions are starting to brown around the edges, and a thermometer inserted in the thickest part of the chicken reads 165 degrees f, 5 to 10 minutes more.
15) Garnish with lemon slices and parsley if you want.
16) Serve and enjoy.

Whole Wheat Spaghetti And Meatballs

Cook Time:
30 minute

Prep Time:
12 minutes

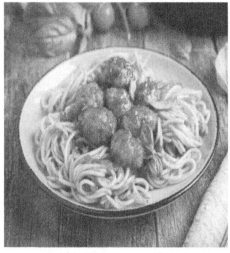

Serving Size
1
Calories per serving:
513kcal
Carbs per serving:
53g

Start with the healthy ingredient like whole-wheat spaghetti to whip up an improved classic Whole Wheat Spaghetti and Meatballs. I mixed Parmesan cheese and ground flaxseed with ground turkey for tasty and healthy meatballs.

Per Serving:

Fat: 20.6g | **Saturated fat:** 4.5g
Protein: 35g | **Fiber:** 11g |
Sodium: 431mg | **Calcium:**
118mg | **Sugar:** 118mg

Tip:

You will enjoy this recipe when served immediately.

Ingredients:

- 2 ounces of whole-wheat spaghetti
- 1/2 teaspoon of kosher salt, divided
- 1 tablespoon of extra-virgin olive oil, divided
- 2.5 garlic cloves, minced
- 1 pound ripe tomatoes, roughly chopped
- 1/2 pound of ground turkey
- 1 tablespoon of ground flax-seed
- 1 tablespoon of freshly grated Parmesan cheese
- 1/2 large egg, lightly beaten
- 0.25 teaspoon of black pepper
- 0.25 teaspoon of crushed red pepper (or to taste)

Direction:

1. Cook the pasta according to the label direction.
2. Reserve 1-1/2 tablespoons of cooking liquid; drain.
3. Meanwhile, combine the turkey, Parmesan, flax-seed, pepper, egg, and 0.25 teaspoon of salt in a large bowl.
4. Mix well and then shape into 4 equal meatballs.
5. In a large skillet over medium heat, heat 1/2 tablespoon of oil.
6. In a single layer, arrange the meatballs in the skillet, working in batches if necessary. Gently cook, turning the meatballs occasionally, for about 10 minutes, just until golden brown on all sides. In the same skillet, heat the other oil and reduce the heat to low. Add the garlic and cook, stirring, for about 2 minutes, until aromatic and golden.
7. Add the crushed red pepper and tomatoes. Stir until well combined. Raise the heat to medium-high.
8. Add the rest of the salt and browned meatballs. Cook, occasionally stirring for about 10 minutes, until the sauce thickens slightly and meatballs are cooked through.
9. Add the reserved cooking liquid and pasta to the meatballs mixture.
10. Toss gently until well combined.
11. Serve hot and enjoy.

Grilled Chicken With Spinach And Butternut

Cook Time:
20 minutes

Prep Time:
15 minutes

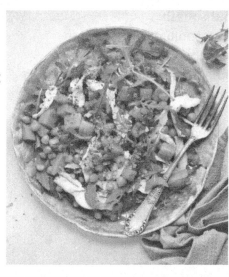

Serving Size
1

**Calories
per serving:**
488kcal

**Carbs
per serving:**
47g

This dinner recipe is a One Pan meal your whole family will enjoy! Grilled Chicken With Spinach and Butternut is your ultimate comfort food recipe idea you need to try tonight. You'll enjoy it for sure.

Per Serving:

Fat: 20g | **Saturated fat:** 4g
Protein: 31g | **Fiber:** 5g |
Sodium: 731mg | **Calcium:**
195mg | **Potassium:** 154mg |
Sugar: 4g

Tip:

Sprinkle this dish evenly with cheese and enjoy.

Ingredients:

- 1-1/2 tablespoons of olive oil, divided
- 1/2 pound of boneless, skinless chicken thighs, cut into 1-in. pieces
- 1/2 butternut squash
- 1/1 cup of low-sodium chicken broth
- 1 teaspoon of chopped fresh sage
- 2 ounces of baby spinach, roughly chopped
- 1 tablespoon of refrigerated prepared pesto
- 1 teaspoon of white wine vinegar
- 3/4 ounces of Parmesan cheese, finely grated
- 1/2 sliced cremini mushrooms
- 1/2 yellow onion, chopped
- 1/2 garlic cloves, chopped
- 1/2 tablespoons of water
- 6 ounces potato gnocchi

Direction:

1) In a large skillet over medium-high, heat 1/2 tablespoon of the oil and add the chicken.
2) Cook, occasionally stirring until cooked through and browned, for about 6 minutes. Transfer into a large bowl.
3) In the skillet over medium-high, heat 1/2 tablespoon of the oil. Add mushrooms, squash, onion, and garlic; cook, occasionally stirring, for about 10 minutes, until just tender.
4) Add water if you want, 1 tablespoon at a time, and stir to loosen browned bits from the bottom of the skillet.
5) Transfer the squash mixture to the bowl with chicken.
6) In the skillet over medium-high, heat the rest of the oil and add the gnocchi, then cook, occasionally stirring, for about 1 minute, until lightly browned. Stir in sage, broth, and chicken mixture. Cover and reduce heat to medium. Cook until most of the liquid is absorbed, and gnocchi is tender, for about 4 minutes. Stir in pesto, spinach, and vinegar; cook, often stirring, for about 1 minute, until spinach is wilted.
7) Sprinkle servings evenly with cheese. Serve and enjoy!

Pan-Seared Trout With Stir-Fried Vegetables

Cook Time:
0 minute

Prep Time:
25 minutes

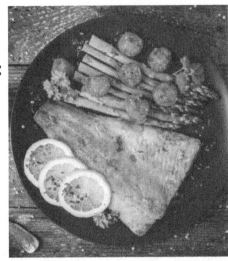

Serving Size
1
Calories per serving:
120kcal
Carbs per serving:
1.6g

The most interesting part of this recipe is that you could certainly use any other kind of fish here. The trout is nice because the filets are so thin that they take just minutes to cook. A thicker fish would take more time to cook through.

Per Serving:

Fat: 12.9g | **Saturated fat:** 4.7g
Protein: 0.5g | **Fiber:** 0.3g |
Sodium: 201mg | **Calcium:** 16mg
| **Potassium:** 56mg | **Sugar:** 0.2g

Tip:

You can add some more butter to the pan after removing the cooked fillets, add some white wine & make a beurre blanc sauce.

Ingredients:

- 1 skin-on trout fillets
- 1 garlic cloves, minced
- 1-1/2 tablespoons of chopped fresh parsley
- 1/2 tablespoon of lemon juice
- 1/2 tablespoon of olive oil
- 1/2 tablespoon of unsalted butter
- salt and pepper, to taste

Direction:

1. Heat a non-stick skillet over medium-high heat.
2. Melt olive oil and butter until frothy.
3. Cook trout fillets for about 2 minutes, skin side down, then carefully use a thin wide spatula to flip.
4. Cook for another minute, until almost cooked through, then add parsley, garlic, and lemon juice.
5. Go ahead with cooking for another minute until the fish is golden brown, and until you can use a fork to fall off the flesh flakes easily.
6. Transfer to the serving plate.
7. Serve yourself and enjoy it.

Beef Strips Stir-Fried Vegetables

Cook Time:
15 minutes

Prep Time:
5 minutes

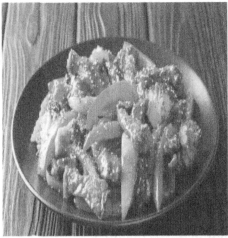

Serving Size
1

Calories per serving:
123kcal

Carbs per serving:
6g

Beef Strips Stir-Fried Vegetables are a quick and easy meal to prepare for dinner. The beef loin is maintained consistency and full of excellent flavor.

Per Serving:

Fat: 3g | **Saturated fat:** 1g
Protein: 18g | **Fiber:** 1g |
Sodium: 283mg | **Sugar:** 0g

Tip:

You can serve this beef alone or over brown rice, baked potato, or pasta.

Ingredients:

- Cooking spray
- 1-1/2 tablespoons of lite teriyaki sauce (58% less sodium)
- 6 ounces of beef tenderloin or filet mignon, cut into bite-size pieces
- 1/2 package (8 ounces) of frozen, mixed, stir-fry blend vegetables, thawed

Direction:

1) Use cooking spray to coat a large non-skillet and warm over medium heat.
2) Add the meat and cook, frequently stirring, for about 4 to 5 minutes, until browned.
3) Increase heat to high. Stir in teriyaki sauce and vegetables.
4) Cook, until vegetables are crisp-tender and meat is heated through, for about 4 to 6 minutes.
5) Stir frequently.
6) Serve alone or over brown rice, baked potato, or pasta.
7) Enjoy!

Fish Tacos With Salad

Cook Time:
45 minutes

Prep Time:
5 minutes

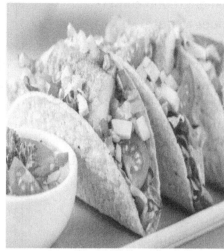

Serving Size
1

Calories per serving:
245kcal

Carbs per serving:
20g

Are you a lover of seafood? This Fish Tacos Salad is healthy with quickly-seared white fish packed with many fresh vegetables. I'm a fan of taco, and I always see a taco of any kind at any time.

Per Serving:

Fat: 6g | **Saturated fat:** 1g
Protein: 25g | **Fiber:** 3g |
Sodium: 335mg | **Sugar:** 4g

Tip:

You might want to leave the sour cream out of the sauce. It's up to you.

Ingredients:

- 1/2 teaspoon of chili powder
- 1/4 teaspoon of ground cumin
- salt and pepper to taste
- 2 teaspoons of olive oil
- 2 limes, juiced
- 2 garlic cloves, minced
- 1 tablespoon of minced cilantro
- 1 teaspoon of hot sauce
- 1 pound of mahimahi or orange roughly fish fillets
- 4 (6-inch) whole-wheat or corn tortillas, warmed
- **Sauce:**
- 2 tablespoons of minced cilantro
- 1 tablespoon of canned green chilies
- 1 cup of chopped cabbage
- pepper to taste
- 1/3 cup of nonfat sour cream or nonfat Greek yogurt
- 1/4 cup of diced fresh avocado
- 1 small tomato, diced
- 1/4 cup of red onion, diced

Direction:

1. Combine the garlic, lime juice, cilantro, and hot sauce in a medium bowl.
2. Add the fish and turn to coat. Let the fish marinate for 30-min in the refrigerator, turning once after 15-min.
3. Remove the fish from the marinade. Pat slightly dry and add cumin, chili powder, salt, and pepper.
4. In a large nonstick skillet, heat the oil and add the fish.
5. Cook per side for about 4 minutes, or until cooked through and tender. Remove the fish from the pan and cut into bite-sized pieces. Add all the sauce ingredients together.
6. Divide the fish among the warmed tortillas.
7. Top with the sauce and fold over the sides to form a taco to eat. Enjoy.

Steak And Sautéed Zucchini

Cook Time:
30 minutes

Prep Time:
5 minutes

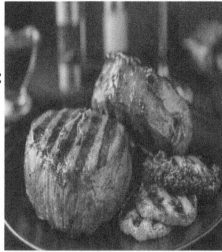

Serving Size
1

Calories per serving:
481kcal

Carbs per serving:
22g

This is a perfect dish for dinner. By the way, having fresh herbs on hand is helpful.

Per Serving:

Fat: 20g | Saturated fat: 5g
Protein: 38g | Fiber: 3g |
Sodium: 342mg | Calcium: 22mg

Tip:

The tip to sautéing zucchini is not to overcook it.

Ingredients:

- 1/2 pound of baby red-skinned potatoes
- 1 teaspoon of chopped fresh thyme
- 1/2 teaspoon of finely grated lemon zest
- 1/2 pound of beef tri-tip, cut lengthwise into 2 steaks
- 1/2 tablespoon of fresh lemon juice
- 1/2 clove garlic, smashed
- Kosher salt
- 1-1/2 tablespoon of extra-virgin olive oil
- 1 teaspoon of chopped fresh rosemary
- 1/2 tablespoon of finely chopped fresh parsley
- Freshly ground pepper
- 2 medium zucchini, sliced diagonally 1 inch thick

Direction:

1) Preheat a grill to medium-high. In a medium saucepan, put the potatoes, and add the 0.25 teaspoon of salt, garlic, and water to cover. Bring to a boil, then reduce the heat to medium-low and simmer, for about 10 minutes, until the potatoes are tender.
2) Drain and discard the garlic.
3) Meanwhile, mix the olive oil, lemon zest, thyme, rosemary, 1/2 teaspoon of salt and pepper to taste in a small bowl.
4) Toss the zucchini in a bowl with 1/2 tablespoon of the herb oil.
5) Use the rest of the herb oil to run the steak.
6) Grill the steak, turning just once until a thermometer inserted into the steak center reads 130 degrees F, about 10 minutes.
7) Transfer to a plate to rest. Meanwhile, grill the zucchini, turning just once, until crisp-tender and well-marked, for about 10 minutes.
8) Transfer to a plate. Sprinkle with half of the lemon juice.
9) Toss the potatoes with the other lemon juice and herb oil, the salt, parsley, and pepper to taste.
10) Serve with the zucchini and steak.
11) Enjoy.

Steak With Sweet Potato And Broccoli

Cook Time:
30 minutes

Prep Time:
5 minutes

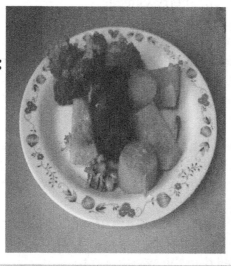

Serving Size
1

Calories per serving:
610kcal

Carbs per serving:
48g

This recipe elevates potatoes and classic steak with a few small touches. A pan sauce made with beef demi-glace which adds rich flavor to the steaks, while the spicy maple syrup adds a hint of heat to the creamy sweet potato mash; this is one of my best diabetic dinner recipes. So you need to try this out.

Per Serving:

Tip:

Fat: 23g | Saturated fat: 11g
Protein: 40g | Fiber: 8g |
Sodium: 400mg | Sugar: 14g

Top the steaks with the pan sauce and enjoy.

Ingredients:

- 2 Steaks
- 1 tablespoon of Spicy Maple Syrup
- 2 tablespoons of Butter
- 1 tablespoon of Sherry Vinegar
- 1/2 pound of Sweet Potatoes
- 1/2 pound of Broccoli
- 1-1/2 tablespoons of Grassfed Beef Demi-Glace

Direction:

1. In the oven center, place an oven rack, and then preheat to 450 degrees F.
2. Heat a medium pot of salted water to a boil on high. Wash and dry the fresh produce.
3. Cut off and discard the bottom of the broccoli stem; cut the broccoli into small florets.
4. Peel and small dice the sweet potatoes.
5. Place the broccoli florets just on a sheet pan and drizzle with 1/2 tablespoon of olive oil, season with pepper and salt; toss to coat.
6. Arrange in an even layer and roast until browned and tender when pierced with a fork. Remove from the oven.
7. While the broccoli roasts, in a pot of boiling water, add the diced sweet potatoes. Cook until tender when pierced with a fork. Then turn off the heat.
8. Thoroughly drain and return to the pot and add half of the butter, spicy maple syrup, and olive oil drizzle. Mash to your desired consistency using a fork; season with pepper and salt to taste. Then cover to keep warm.
9. Pat the steaks dry with paper towels while the sweet potatoes cook.
10. Season with pepper and salt on both sides.
11. Heat olive oil on medium-high in a large pan until hot. Add the seasoned steaks. Cook, occasionally turning for 10 minutes, until cooked to your desired degree of doneness and browned.

Leaving any bits in the pan, transfer to a cutting board. Let it rest for 5 minutes.

12. While the steak rest, add the vinegar, 1/8 cup of water, and demi-glace to the pan of reserved fond. Cook on medium-high, scraping up any fond and occasionally stirring until slightly reduced in volume, for about 3 minutes. Turn off the heat.

13. Stir in the rest of the butter until melted and season with pepper and salt to taste.

14. Find the lines of the muscle on the rested steaks, and slice crosswise against the grain.

15. Serve the steaks with roasted broccoli and mashed sweet potatoes.

16. Top the steaks with the pan sauce and enjoy it.

Fish Tacos With Stir-Fried Vegetables

Cook Time:
10 minutes

Prep Time:
20 minutes

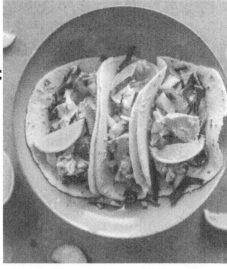

Serving Size
1

Calories per serving:
435.99kcal

Carbs per serving:
34.98g

This kind of fish taco is a class by itself.

Per Serving:

Fat: 15.4g | Saturated fat: 3.13g
Protein: 39.71g | Fiber: 2.72g |
Sodium: 642.13mg | Calcium:
89.74mg | Potassium: 740.23mg
| Sugar: 4.13g

Tip:

Serve the tortillas with the vegetable relish, fish, and along with the queso fresco on the side.

Ingredients:

- 0.13 cucumber peeled, halved lengthwise, seeded, and cut into thin half-moons
- 0.13 red onion cut into wedges, then slivered
- 0.13 cup of chopped fennel
- 0.06 cup of chopped olives optional
- 0.5 tablespoon of fresh lemon juice
- 2 6-inch flour or corn tortillas
- 0.5 tablespoon of olive oil divided
- 1 6-ounce of filet tilapia, cod, barramundi, or other flaky white fish
- 0.13 teaspoon of ground coriander
- 0.13 teaspoon of ground cumin
- Kosher salt with freshly ground pepper, to taste
- 2 radishes quartered and thinly sliced
- Crumbled queso fresco to serve

Direction:

1) The first thing need to do is heat a large nonstick skillet over medium-high heat.
2) Add 1 tablespoon of oil and sprinkle both sides of the fish fillets with the cumin, coriander, salt, and pepper while the oil is heating.
3) Sear the fish until browned and cooked through, for about 3 minutes per side.
4) Transfer the fish onto a plate. Break it into small chunks and tent with foil to keep warm. Wash the skillet out and while the fish is cooking, combine the cucumbers, radishes, red onion, olives(if using), fennel, lemon juice, and the rest of the oil—season with pepper and salt.
5) Return the clean, dry skillet to medium-high heat.
6) Cook the tortillas on each side for flour, 45 seconds on each side until softened and lightly browned in spots. Stack them on a plate.
7) Serve and enjoy.

Hummus And Olive Oil Salad With Cottage Cheese

Cook Time:
0 minute

Prep Time:
15 minutes

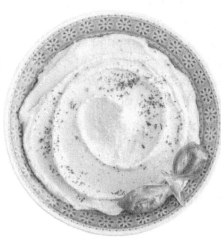

Serving Size
1

Calories per serving:
203kcal

Carbs per serving:
28.79g

The Hummus still has all of the great flavors of this classic dish. The best hummus you can serve up with crispy and fresh vegetables, for a healthy, diet-friendly treat.

Per Serving:

Fat: 5.62g | Saturated fat: 0.88g
Protein: 10.58g | Fiber: 5.56g |
Sodium: 528.72mg | Calcium:
147.5mg | Potassium: 283.80mg
| Sugar: 0.90g

Tip:

Serve with pita bread or fresh vegetables.

Ingredients:

- 1/2 cup of 1% low-fat cottage cheese
- 2 tablespoons of tahini
- 1/8 teaspoon of salt
- 1 clove garlic
- One (15 ounces) can of garbanzo beans, drain & save liquid (then rinse & drain)
- 1/4 cup of fresh parsley, chopped finely
- 1/4 teaspoon of grated lemon rind
- 1 tablespoon of freshly squeezed lemon juice
- 1/2 teaspoon of ground coriander
- fresh veggies or pita, for serving

Direction:

1. Place all the ingredients except pita/veggies and parsley in a food processor; process until smooth.
2. Use reserved garbanzo bean liquid to thin out the hummus.
3. Taste and adjust spices if you want.
4. Stir in the parsley.
5. Scoop the hummus into a dish. Cover and store in the refrigerator.
6. Serve with fresh vegetables and pita bread.
   Enjoy.

Soups Recipes

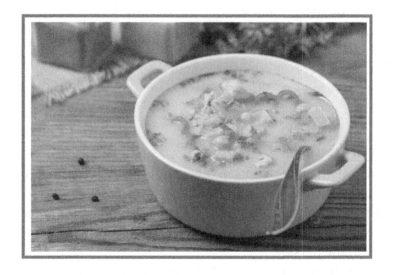

Slow-Cooker Chicken Noodle Soup

Cook Time:
7 hours

Prep Time:
15 minutes

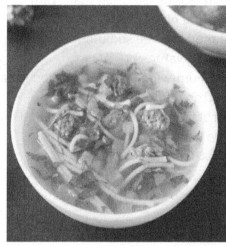

Serving Size
1

Calories per serving:
357.4kcal

Carbs per serving:
23.2g

This is a soup that is such easy and great comfort food! You'll love the mushrooms and the addition of spinach. Have a taste of this Diabetic great soup.

Per Serving:

Fat: 18.7g | Saturated fat: 5.3g
Protein: 23.9g | Fiber: 3.1g |
Sodium: 134.4mg | Sugar: 3.2g

Tip:

Add cooked noodles to the soup just before serving, and season with pepper and salt.

Ingredients:

- 1 (3/8 pound) whole chickens, cut into 8 pieces
- 1/4 large onions (one should be peeled and quartered and one should be small diced)
- 1/16 teaspoon of crushed dried marjoram
- 1/16 fresh ground black pepper
- 1/8 quart canned fat-free sodium-free chicken broth
- 1/8 quart boiling water
- 3/4 ounce medium-wide noodles (cooked separately)
- 1/2 ounce button of mushrooms, sliced
- 3/8 large carrots (one should be peeled and quartered and two should be small diced)
- 3/8 sprig of flat-leaf parsley
- 1/16 teaspoon of crushed dried thyme
- 1/16 pound of fresh spinach, well washed and large stems removed
- 1/4 stalk celery & leaves, and diced small

Direction:

1) Rinse and pat dry the chicken—place in a larger crockery slow cooker. Place the quartered and peeled onion, carrot, and parsley around the chicken pieces. Then sprinkle with marjoram, thyme, and pepper.
2) Add chicken broth, cover, and cook on low for about 7 hours or high for 3 hours. Remove the chicken when done cooking and discard the carrot, parsley, and onion.
3) Skim off and discard all surface fat from the broth.
4) Cool chicken from broth back to the slow-cooker, then bring to a simmer. Saute the diced carrots, onion, celery, and mushroom lightly, in a little water until softened and place in the crock along with the spinach. Simmer for about 10 minutes.
5) Meanwhile, cook the noodles according to the package direction.
6) Just before serving, add cooked noodles to the soup.
7) Season with pepper and salt to taste. Serve and enjoy.

Tomato Soup

Cook Time:
20 minutes

Prep Time:
15 minutes

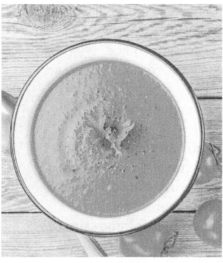

Serving Size
1

Calories per serving:
94kcal

Carbs per serving:
13g

This kind of Tomato soup is a healthy and tasty recipe for a classic! As its name suggests, mainly tomato with a mixture of some additional ingredients for taste. If you're sourcing local tomatoes, look for ones that are not too hard or sour. You could go for canned tomatoes as well.

Per Serving:

Fat: 2g | **Saturated fat:** 0.3g
Protein: 7g | **Fiber:** 1g | **Sodium:** 112mg | **Sugar:** 0g

Tip:

Do not let the mixture boil after stirring in the evaporated milk.

Ingredients:

- 1 tablespoon of reduced-fat margarine
- 1 tablespoon of canola oil
- 3 14.5-ounce cans of no-salt-added diced tomatoes with the juice
- 5 cups of no-salt-added canned chicken broth
- pinch cayenne pepper (optional)
- salt (optional)
- 1 medium onion, finely chopped
- 1/2 teaspoon of crushed dried thyme
- 1/4 teaspoon of crushed dried oregano
- freshly ground pepper (to taste)
- 2 12-ounce cans of evaporated skim milk

Direction:

1. Heat margarine and oil over medium heat in a heavy soup pot.
2. Add onion and cook, frequently stirring, for about 10 minutes, until onion is very limp, taking care to not let the onion brown.
3. Add oregano, thyme, tomatoes with their juices and chicken broth.
4. Bring to a boil. Reduce heat to low. Simmer, partially covered for about 20 minutes.
5. Taste soup, adding salt, cayenne, and pepper.
6. Stir in evaporated milk and heat through - make sure the mixture is not actually boiling.
7. Serve and enjoy.

Creamy Asparagus Soup

Cook Time:
10 minutes

Prep Time:
15 minutes

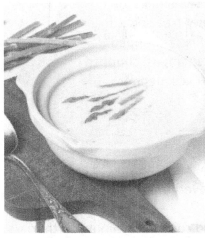

Serving Size
1

Calories per serving:
151kcal

Carbs per serving:
14.0g

This kind of Creamy Asparagus Soup is a tasty dairy-free version using soya milk and perfect for diabetic people.

Per Serving:

Fat: 8.2g | Saturated fat: 3.30g
Protein: 20.7g | Fiber: 3.1g |
Sugar: 9.8g

Tip:

Soup keeps, covered and chilled, 2 days.

Ingredients:

- 25 grams of plain flour
- 450milliltre of vegetable stock
- 150millilitre of soya milk
- 15 grams of dairy-free spread
- 1 small onion, finely chopped
- 125 grams of asparagus, chopped
- freshly ground black pepper

Direction:

1) In a medium pan, heat the spread and add the asparagus and onion. Fry until everything starts to soften, for about 2o to 3 minutes.
2) Add the flour and cook for a minute further.
3) Stir in the stock gradually and bring to the boil. Simmer until the asparagus is cooked through, for about 10 minutes, and reserve a couple of asparagus spears for serving.
4) Add the milk. Bring to an almost boiling point, then place in a food processor and blend until smooth.
5) Season with lots of black pepper.
6) Top with the asparagus spears.
7) Serve with crusty toast or bread.
8) Enjoy.

Coconut Chicken Soup

Cook Time:

30 minutes

Prep Time:

20 minutes

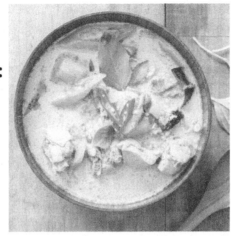

Serving Size

1

Calories per serving:

231kcal

Carbs per serving:

11.6g

This rich aroma and taste of this easy Coconut Chicken Soup will warm your soul and belly. It's packed with lean chicken breast and vegetables. This dish will keep you satisfied and full for hours. I hope you enjoy it as well.

Per Serving:

Fat: 12.7g | **Saturated fat:** 5.5g
Protein: 17.1g | **Fiber:** 1.7g |
Sodium: 45.1mg | **Calcium:** 19mg
| **Potassium:** 357.5mg | **Sugar:**
5g

Tip:

This dish reheats very well. You can store in an airtight container in the refrigerator for up to 3 to 4 days if you have leftovers.

Ingredients:

- 0.17 pound of chicken breast, thinly sliced
- Salt & pepper, to taste
- 0.13 pound of pumpkin, cubed into 1/2 inch pieces (1 cup)
- 0.17 red bell pepper, seeds removed and thinly sliced
- 0.17 small chili or jalapeño pepper, seeds removed and thinly sliced
- 2.33 ounces of lite coconut milk (1 can)
- 0.33 cups of chicken broth
- 0.17 tablespoon of coconut oil (or vegetable oil)
- 0.17 small onion, thinly sliced into half-moons
- 0.33 garlic cloves, minced
- 0.17-inch piece ginger, peeled and minced
- 0.17 medium zucchini, cut into quarters lengthwise and diced
- Juice of 1 lime
- Handful cilantro leaves (optional)

Direction:

1. Season the sliced chicken breast generously with pepper and salt. Heat the coconut oil in a large soup pot over high heat and add the chicken breast. Stir-fry over high until the chicken is no longer pink on the outside, for about 4 to 5 minutes. Add the minced garlic, sliced onion, and minced ginger.
2. Continue to stir-fry for another 2 to 3 minutes.
3. Ass the cubed pumpkin and zucchini, then stir.
4. Add the sliced chili or jalapeno pepper, sliced bell pepper, coconut milk, lime juice, and chicken broth - give everything another stir.
5. Bring to a boil and then low the heat. Cover and allow to simmer until the pumpkin is fully cooked for about 20 minutes.
6. Remove from the heat and season with additional pepper and salt, if you want. Garnish with cilantro leaves to serve.
7. Enjoy.

Sweet Potato And Chicken Soup

Cook Time:
20 minutes

Prep Time:
10 minutes

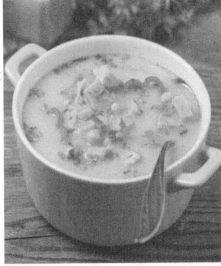

Serving Size
1

Calories per serving:
1773kcal

Carbs per serving:
50g

Enjoy this Immune-boosting soup for lunch loaded with sweet potato and turmeric. You can top with parsley if you'll be using it. What an easy soup recipe that is quick and delicious at the same time!

Per Serving:

Fat: 10.3g | Saturated fat: 3.5g
Protein: 30.5g | Fiber: 4.4g |
Sugar: 0g

Tip:

You can serve soup topped with parsley.

Ingredients:

- 1 Massel chicken style stock cube
- 55grams (1/3 cup) of roasted sweet potato
- 45grams (1/4 cup) of canned chickpeas, rinsed, drained
- 20grams of baby spinach
- 200grams of chicken breast
- 400grams packet of Hart & Soul Sweet Potato Ginger Soup with Turmeric
- Fresh continental parsley leaves, to serve (optional)

Direction:

1) In the saucepan, bring 3 cups of water to boil.
2) Add the stock cube and stir until dissolved, then add chicken.
3) Reduce heat to low, cover, and cook until just cooked through, for about 15 minutes.
4) Remove from the heat and set aside in the pan for about 5-min. Transfer to a plate.
5) Halve the poached chicken. Use half in the soup and reserve the rest for another use.
6) Heat the soup following the packet direction. And shred chicken.
7) Stir through soup with chickpeas, sweet potato, and spinach until warmed.
8) Microwave again, if you want, and season.
9) Serve soup topped with parsley, if you'll be using.
10) Enjoy.

Pasta And Bean Soup

Cook Time:
30 minutes

Prep Time:
10 minutes

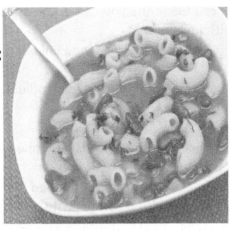

Serving Size
1

Calories per serving:
191kcal

Carbs per serving:
35g

Pasta and beans may not sound enticing, but I assure you that this stew is genuinely irresistible. It's packed with lots of aromatics, freshly ground pepper, tomatoes, mushroom, zucchini, and Parmesan cheese, which turns pasta and beans into a hearty meal in a bowl situation.

Per Serving:

Fat: 2g | Saturated fat: 0.5g
Protein: 9g | Fiber: 4g | Sodium: 181mg | Sugar: 0g

Tip:

Top with a sprinkling of Parmesan cheese, just before serving and enjoy!

Ingredients:

- 2 ounces (60 grams) button mushrooms, cleaned and sliced
- 1 14 1/2-ounce (435 grams) no-salt-added diced tomatoes with juice
- 1 16-ounce (480 grams) can of cannellini beans, rinsed well
- 3 cups (720 ml) of canned fat-free low-sodium beef or vegetable broth freshly ground pepper
- olive oil cooking spray
- 1 small onion, 4 ounces (120 grams), chopped
- 1 carrot, 3 ounces (90 grams), chopped
- 1 zucchini, 4 ounces (120 grams), chopped
- 6 ounces (180 grams) dried penne pasta or other pasta
- 2 tablespoons (24 grams) of grated Parmesan cheese

Direction:

1. Use cooking spray to spray a nonstick covered pot.
2. Add the carrot, onion, mushrooms, and zucchini; saute until onions wilt, for about 5 to 6 minutes.
3. Add the tomatoes with their juice. Simmer, covered, for about 20 minutes.
4. Add the beans, simmer, uncovered, for about 5 minutes.
5. Add the broth and cook, but uncovered, for about 10 minutes.
6. Cool and freeze in an airtight container.
7. Reheat in a pot or in the microwave when ready to serve.
8. Cook the pasta according to the package direction while the soup is reheating - do not overcook the pasta, or else, it'll continue to cook in the hot soup).
9. Drain the pasta and combine it with the soup.
10. Ladle into soup bowls, and top each serving with a sprinkling of Parmesan cheese.
11. Serve and enjoy.

Dessert
Recipes

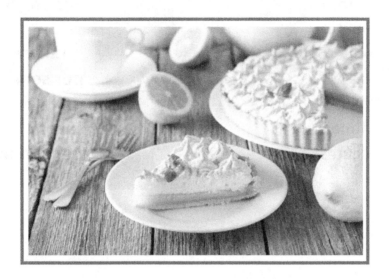

No-Added Sugar Strawberry Shortcake

Cook Time:
10 minutes

Prep Time:
15 minutes

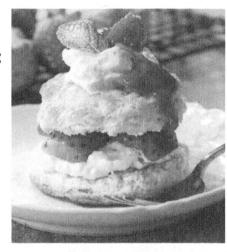

Serving Size
1

Calories per serving:
82kcal

Carbs per serving:
16g

This recipe is a no-added-sugar strawberry shortcake layered with ripe berries and silky whipped cream. Each tender biscuits is made with whole wheat flour & three simple components; it's an easy
dessert with stunning gourmet results.

Per Serving:

Fat: 1g | **Saturated fat:** 0.2g
Protein: 2g | **Fiber:** 2g | **Sodium:** 159mg | **Sugar:** 0g

Tip:

Top your shortcake with strawberry and half tablespoon of the whipped topping.

Ingredients:

- 1 cup of skim milk
- 1 packet of artificial sweetener
- 6 cups of sliced fresh strawberries
- refrigerated butter-flavored cooking spray
- 1 -1/4 cups of low-fat biscuit and baking mix
- 12 tablespoons of fat-free, no sugar added frozen whipped topping, thawed

Direction:

1) Preheat the oven to 400 degrees F.
2) Coat a nonstick baking sheet lightly using cooking spray.
3) Combine the milk, biscuit mix, and sweetener in a bowl, mixing until just combined.
4) Roll dough out on a floured surface into a circle 1/3-inch thick.
5) Cut out 6 biscuits using a 2-inch biscuit cutter, reusing scraps as needed.
6) On your prepared baking sheet, place the biscuits.
7) Spray the tops of the biscuits lightly using cooking spray and bake until nicely browned and done, for about 10 minutes.
8) Split the biscuits in half horizontally, placing half in each of 12 dessert dishes.
9) Top each with 1/2 cup of strawberries and 1 tablespoon of whipped topping.
10) Serve immediately and enjoy it.

Carrot-Cake

Cook Time:
45 minutes

Prep Time:
20 minutes

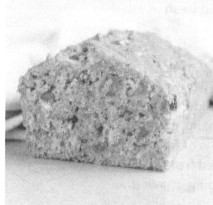

Serving Size
1

Calories per serving:
103kcal

Carbs per serving:
19g

The carrot itself makes this carrot cake a healthy dessert. It's so fluffy, soft, and sweet. It's sugar-free, 100% whole grain, and it's delicious!

Per Serving:

Fat: 2g | **Saturated fat:** 0.2g
Protein: 3g | **Fiber:** 1g | **Sodium:**
123mg | **Sugar:** 0g

Tip:

Slide your knife around and the center of the cake. This will help in loosing it from the pan.

Ingredients:

- cooking spray
- 2 teaspoons of baking powder
- 1/2 teaspoon of baking soda
- 1/4 teaspoon of salt
- 1 teaspoon of ground cinnamon
- 1/2 teaspoon of ground nutmeg
- 1 cup of shredded carrots
- 2 large egg whites, at room temperature
- 1/2 cup of plain non-fat yogurt
- 3 tablespoons of canola oil
- 3/4 cup of unsweetened applesauce
- 1/3 cup of dark brown sugar, packed
- 2 teaspoons of vanilla extract
- 2-1/2 cups of all-purpose flour
- 4 ounces of unsweetened crushed pineapple with juice
- 1/4 cup of dark raisins
- 1/4 cup of sugar substitute

Direction:

1. Preheat the oven to 400 degrees F. Position the top rack in the center of the oven. Coat a 9-inch cake pan lightly using cooking spray. Dust with flour, then tap out excess. Whisk together yogurt, oil, egg whites, brown sugar, applesauce, vanilla, pineapple with juice in a large bowl.
2. Sift together the baking powder, salt (if using), baking soda, flour, nutmeg, and cinnamon in a bowl.
3. Add to egg-applesauce mixture gradually, stirring until the cake batter. Spoon the batter into the prepared pan, smoothing the top using the back of a spoon. Bake until a toothpick inserted in the center comes out clean, for about 30 to 40 minutes.
4. Cool in the pan on a rack for 10-min.
5. Slide a thin knife just around the edges to loosen the cake from the pan. Invert onto a rack to cool. Transfer cake into a serving platter when ready to serve. Serve and enjoy.

Brownie Sundae Pie

Cook Time:
20 minutes

Prep Time:
15 minutes

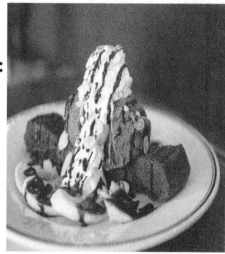

Serving Size
1
**Calories
per serving:**
150kcal
**Carbs
per serving:**
28g

Brownie Sundae Pie is so descendent, but worth every bite! You're going to want this pie for your next birthday!Serve with non-fat frozen vanilla yogurt!

Per Serving:

Fat: 4g | **Saturated fat:** 1.0g
Protein: 2g | **Fiber:** 0g | **Sodium:** 160mg

Tip:

Serve with a non-fat frozen vanilla yogurt. Also, the nutritional information in this recipe is based on the recipe without the non-fat yogurt.

Ingredients:

- 1/2 teaspoon of baking powder
- 1/8 teaspoon of salt
- 1/2 cup of reduced-calories frozen whipped topping, thawed
- 1/2 cups of sliced bananas
- 2 tablespoons of chopped walnuts
- cooking spray
- 2/3 cup of sugar
- 6 tablespoons of reduced-calorie margarine, melted
- 1 large egg
- 1 teaspoon of vanilla extract
- 1/2 cup of all-purpose flour
- 1/3 cup of unsweetened cocoa powder
- 1 -1/2 cups of non-fat vanilla frozen yogurt (optional)

Direction:

1) Preheat oven to 350 degrees F.
2) Spray a 9-inch pie pan with cooking spray.
3) Combine the margarine, sugar, vanilla, and egg until well blended in a large bowl.
4) Stir in the cocoa, flour, salt, and baking powder until well incorporated.
5) Spread in the prepared pan. Bake for about 20 minutes.
6) Cool on a wire rack completely.
7) Spoon the whipped topping decoratively around the edges of the pie just before serving.
8) Garnish with walnuts and banana slices.
9) Cut the pie into 8 wedges. Serve with non-fat frozen vanilla yogurt if you want.
10) Enjoy.

Lemon Meringue Pie

Cook Time:
15 minutes

Prep Time:
30 minutes

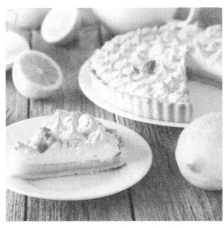

Serving Size
1
Calories per serving:
153kcal
Carbs per serving:
14g

You need to try this diabetes-friendly version of a tangy and classic dessert like this. The result will wow you! This is a beautiful recipe that calls for vanilla extract, lemon zest, yellow food coloring, and the cream of tartar.

Per Serving:

Fat: 9g | **Saturated fat:** 2.0g
Protein: 3g | **Fiber:** 0g | **Sodium:** 152mg

Tip:

Make sure you cool before serving, and you can refrigerate leftovers for no more than 2 days.

Ingredients:

- 1 cup of SugarTwin® Spoonable
- 1 teaspoon of grated lemon zest
- 3 large eggs, separated
- 2 drops of yellow food coloring (optional)
- 1 9-inch fresh or frozen pie shell, baked and cooled
- 1/4 teaspoon of cream of tartar
- 1/2 pure vanilla extract
- 1/2 cup of cornstarch
- 1/4 teaspoon of cream of tartar
- 1/4 teaspoon of salt
- 1-1/2 cups of water
- 1/2 cup of fresh lemon juice
- 2 tablespoons of margarine

Direction:

1) Combine cream of tartar, salt, cornstarch, 1 cup of SugarTwin in a nonstick medium saucepan. Whisk in lemon juice and water.
2) Cook over medium heat and stir until the mixture boils. Reduce heat to medium-low. Go ahead with cooking and stirring for a minute.
3) Remove from heat. Stir in lemon zest and margarine; set it aside.
4) Whisk together egg yolks until lemon-colored in a medium bowl.
5) Whisk at least half of the hot cornstarch mixture into eggs. Stir this mixture into the rest of the mixture in saucepan, blending well.
6) Return pan to medium-low heat. Cook, stirring, for about 2 minutes.
7) Slightly cool and pour filling into a baked pie crust—Preheat oven to 350 degrees F.

Making the Meringue:

8) Combine egg whites and 1/4 teaspoon of cream of tartar in a small bowl.

9) Beat with an electric mixer until froth on high-speed. Add vanilla. Gradually add SugarTwin, and one tablespoon at a time. Beat until it stiff peaks form.

10) Evenly spread over lemon filling, sealing well around the edge of the crust.

11) Swirl peaks by lifting up some of the meringue with the back of a spoon if you want.

12) Bake until meringue is golden brown, for about 15 minutes.

13) Cool before serving.

14) Refrigerate leftover for no more than two days.

15) Serve and enjoy.

Banana Chocolate Parfaits

Cook Time:
0 minute

Prep Time:
10 minutes

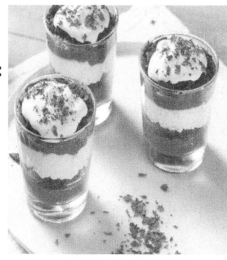

Serving Size
1

Calories per serving:
138kcal

Carbs per serving:
25g

This is a creamy combination of sugar-free chocolate pudding mix and frozen dairy whipped topping, with low-fat yogurt.

Per Serving:

Fat: 3g | **Saturated fat:** 1.3g
Protein: 4g | **Fiber:** 2g | **Sodium:** 336mg

Tip:

Sprinkle with walnuts and you can add a raspberry on top, if using.

Ingredients:

- 1 cup of plain low-fat yogurt
- 1/4 cup of reduced-fat frozen dairy whipped topping
- unsweetened cocoa powder
- 1 tablespoon of chopped walnuts (optional)
- 1 0.8-ounce box of sugar-free chocolate pudding mix
- 2 medium bananas
- 1 teaspoon of fresh lemon juice
- 4 fresh raspberries (for garnish)

Direction:

1. Fold in yogurt.
2. Cut each banana into six pieces on the diagonal.
3. Sprinkle with lemon juice.
4. Place two bananas quarters in each of 4 parfait glasses.
5. Top with 1/4 of the pudding mix.
6. Top each with one tablespoon of whipped topping.
7. Sift a little cocoa powder on top of each serving using a fine sieve.
8. Sprinkle with walnuts.
9. Add a raspberry too if you want.
10. Enjoy.

Sliced Baked Apples

Cook Time:
30 minutes

Prep Time:
5 minutes

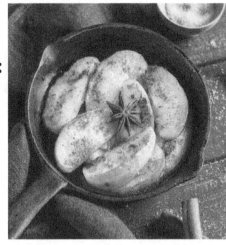

Serving Size
1

Calories per serving:
118kcal

Carbs per serving:
29g

These Sliced Baked Apples are low in sugar and delicious enough for dessert. They are perfectly nutritious.

Per Serving:

Fat: 1g | **Saturated fat:** 0.1g
Protein: 1g | **Fiber:** 5g | **Sodium:** 1mg

Tip:

Top with 1/4 of the walnuts.

Ingredients:

- 1/3 cup of unsweetened apple juice
- 1/3 cup of dry white wine
- 1/3 cup of water
- 2 tablespoons of grated orange zest
- 4 medium-size, 6 ounces each, baking apples
- ground cinnamon to taste
- 1 tablespoon of ground walnuts

Direction:

1) Preheat oven to 375 degrees F.
2) Simmer the apple juice, water, and wine with the orange zest in a small pot, for about 10 minutes.
3) Meanwhile, core the apples and remove peel from the top 1/3 of each apple.
4) Remove and discard the seed and core using a small spoon.
5) In a small baking dish, place them just big enough for the apples.
6) Pout apple juice mixture around the apples. Sprinkle cinnamon on each of the apples.
7) Bake until the apples are cooked through, for about 20 minutes, but still, hold their shape.
8) Place each of the apples in a small dessert dish.
9) Top with one tablespoon of the cooking liquid with 1/4 of the walnuts.
10) Serve warm and enjoy.

Snacks &
Biscuits
Recipes

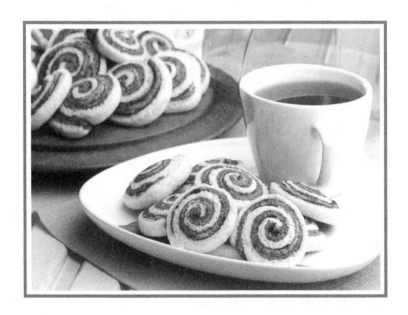

Chocolate Chip Cookies

Cook Time:
10 minutes

Prep Time:
10 minutes

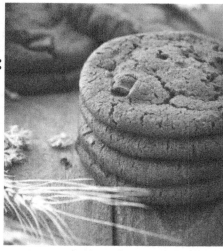

Serving Size
1

Calories per serving:
50kcal

Carbs per serving:
5g

Chocolate Chip Cookies are made with two kinds of cocoa powder for a deep chocolate flavor. These cookies feature brownie-like centers, soft and crisp edges.
They are studded with chocolate and sprinkled with salt to taste.

Per Serving:

Fat: 3g | Saturated fat: 0.8g
Protein: 1g | Fiber: 0g | Sodium: 50mg | Calcium: 0mg

Tip:

The secret of this recipe is the soft butter. Make sure you don't put it in the batter directly from refrigerator, just soft, and don't let it melt.

Ingredients:

- 1/2 cup (1 stick) of softened margarine or butter
- 1/4 cup of sugar
- 3 tablespoons of cocoa powder
- 1/2 teaspoon of baking soda
- 1/8 teaspoon of salt
- 2 tablespoons of skim milk
- sugar substitute equal to 1/2 cup of sugar
- 1 large egg
- 1 teaspoon of vanilla extract
- 1 cup of flour
- 1/3 cup of semi-sweet chocolate chips

Direction:

1. Preheat oven to 375 degrees F.
2. Beat sugar, butter, and sugar substitute in a medium bowl, until well blended.
3. Add vanilla and egg; then beat until combined.
4. Sift together cocoa powder, flour, salt, and baking soda.
5. Alternately add flour and milk mixture to butter and sugar mixture, beating until well blended between additions.
6. Stir in chocolate chips.
7. Drop by teaspoonfuls onto the ungreased cookie sheet. Press flat and bake until set, for about 7 minutes.
8. Remove from cookie sheet to wire rack.
9. Cool completely, serve, and enjoy.

Baked Pita Chips

Cook Time:
5 minutes

Prep Time:
5 minutes

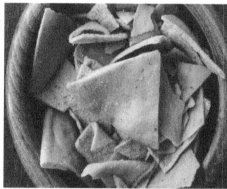

Serving Size
1

Calories per serving:
83kcal

Carbs per serving:
17g

Have you been searching for a good diabetic snack recipe? These chips are amazing baked pita chips you should try today! They are very easy to make, healthy, and they can be served at parties as well. I hope you enjoy the fantastic taste of these chips.

Per Serving:

Fat: 5.2g | **Saturated fat:** 0.8g
Protein: 3g | **Fiber:** 1g | **Sodium:** 161mg

Tip:

You can store in an airtight containers. This recipe is terrific with hummus or guacamole.

Ingredients:

- 6 6-inch pita breads
- cooking spray
- Mrs. Dash or various spices to taste

Direction:

1) Preheat oven to 375 degrees F.
2) Cut each pita bread into 6 wedges with a sharp knife.
3) Pull apart each triangle to separate it into 2 pieces gently, getting 12 triangles per pita bread.
4) In a single layer, lay the triangles on a large non-stick baking sheet. You can use parchment paper if you want.
5) Coat triangles with cooking spray lightly and sprinkle on spices.
6) Bake until pita starts to color, for about 7 minutes.
7) Turn pita over and continue to bake until golden brown and crisp, for about 5 minutes.
8) Store in an airtight container.
9) Serve and enjoy.

Oatmeal Raisin Cookies

Cook Time:
10 minutes

Prep Time:
20 minutes

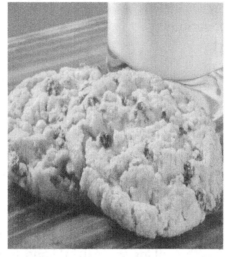

Serving Size
1

**Calories
per serving:**
155kcal

**Carbs
per serving:**
24g

If you often cook diabetes foods at home, then this is one of the great recipes you should go for. Oatmeal Raisin Cookie recipes use rolled oats and are very delicious, easy, and quick.

Per Serving:

Fat: 6g | **Saturated fat:** 1.0g
Protein: 2g | **Fiber:** 1g | **Sodium:** 119mg

Tip:

These Oatmeal Raisin Cookies can be eaten after having your breakfast meal.

Ingredients:

- 1/4 teaspoon of ground cinnamon
- 1/8 teaspoon of salt
- 1/2 cup of margarine (at room temperature)
- 3/4 cup of light brown sugar
- 2 tablespoons of granulated sugar
- 1 large egg
- cooking spray
- 1 cup of unbleached all-purpose flour
- 1/2 teaspoon of baking soda
- 2 tablespoons of 1% milk
- 1/2 teaspoon of vanilla extract
- 1-1/2 cups of rolled oats
- 1/2 cup of dark raisins

Direction:

1. Preheat oven to 350 degrees F.
2. Coat a large cookie sheet using cooking spray.
3. Sift together baking soda, flour, salt, and cinnamon into a bowl. Set it aside.
4. Cream the margarine and sugars until fluffy and light using an electric mixer.
5. Add the milk, egg, and vanilla. Beat well.
6. Add the flour mixture gradually, 1/4 cup at a time, beating after each addition until the flour is incorporated.
7. By hand, stir in rolled raisins and rolled oats.
8. Drop by rounded teaspoonful onto prepared cookie sheet at least 2-inches apart.
9. Bake for about 10 minutes, until golden brown.
10. Transfer cookies to rack to cool.
11. Serve and enjoy.

Vanilla And Chocolate Swirl Cookies

Cook Time:
8 minutes

Prep Time:
3 hr 38 min

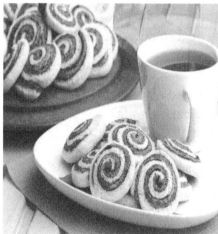

Serving Size
1

Calories per serving:
85kcal

Carbs per serving:
9g

Are you looking for fun cookies to make? These Vanilla and Chocolate Swirl Cookies are enjoyable cookies to make. They are so beautiful, and they look yummy. Having this cookie after eating my dinner would be great!

Per Serving:

Fat: 5g | Saturated fat: 0g
Protein: 2g | Fiber: 0g | Sodium: 73mg

Tip:

Freeze the dough for about 3 hours

Ingredients:

- 1-1/2 cups of unbleached all-purpose flour
- 1/2 teaspoon of baking powder
- 1/4 cup of skim milk, warmed to room temperature
- 1 teaspoon of unsweetened cocoa powder
- 1/8 teaspoon of vanilla extract
- 1/2 cup of margarine, softened
- 2 tablespoons of sugar
- 2 teaspoons of vanilla extract
- 6 tablespoons of liquid egg substitute
- cooking spray

Direction:

1. Cream the margarine, vanilla, sugar, and egg substitute.
2. Add baking powder, flour, and three tablespoons of the milk; stir to mix thoroughly.
3. Divide dough into 2 parts. Add cocoa to one part, stirring until it's well blended. Add vanilla extract to the other half.
4. Chill both halves for at least 60 minutes.
5. Working on a floured surface, roll out each part to a rectangle about 3-inches wide and 18 inches long.
6. On top of the white part, place the chocolate part, pressing together tightly with a rolling pin.
7. Use the remaining milk to brush the chocolate dough. Roll up like a jelly roll to make a log for about 1 to 1/2-inches in diameter.
8. Wrap in waxed paper. Chill for about 2 hours, until firm.
9. Preheat oven to 375 degrees F when you're ready to bake.
10. Slice cookies for about 1/8 inch thick. Place on a non-stick cookie sheet that has been coated with cooking spray.
11. Bake until lightly browned, for about 8 minutes. Transfer to a wire rack to cool.
12. Serve and enjoy.

Raspberry Thumbprint Cookie

Cook Time:
10 minutes

Prep Time:
20 minutes

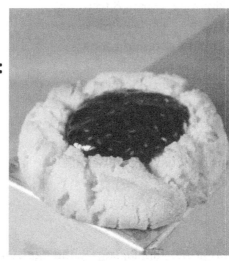

Serving Size
1

Calories per serving:
85kcal

Carbs per serving:
1g

These raspberry imprint cookies are a great combination of flavors. They are simple and delicious.

Per Serving:

Fat: 3g | Saturated fat: 0g
Protein: 1g | Fiber: 0g | Sodium: 43mg

Tip:

Spoon half a teaspoon of the raspberry fruit spread into the center of each cookie, and enjoy!

Ingredients:

- 1 large egg white
- 1 teaspoon of vanilla extract
- 1/4 cup of margarine, softened
- 3 tablespoons of sugar
- 1-1/2 cups of sifted all-purpose flour
- cooking spray
- 3 tablespoons of no-sugar-added raspberry fruit spread

Direction:

1) Preheat oven to 350 degrees F.
2) Cream margarine and sugar until fluffy and light in a large bowl.
3) Add vanilla and egg white. Beat well.
4) Stir in flour in 3 parts, stirring well each time until the flour is well-incorporated.
5) Form dough into a ball using your hands. Wrap in plastic wrap. Then chill for about 30 mins.
6) Shape down into 1-inch balls, and place 2 inches apart on a cookie sheet that has been coated with cooking spray.
7) Press a hole in the center of each cookie using your thumb.
8) Bake until golden for about 10 minutes.
9) Cool completely on wire racks.
10) Spoon half a teaspoon of the raspberry fruit spread into the center of each cookie.
11) Serve and enjoy.

Cranberry Scones

Cook Time:
15 minutes

Prep Time:
10 minutes

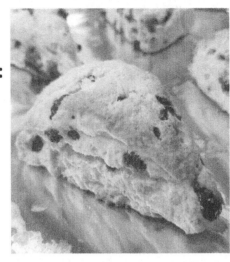

Serving Size
1

Calories per serving:
91kcal

Carbs per serving:
15g

You all know that scones are best eaten fresh out of the oven, right? This Cranberry scones can be your perfect bite to go along with your morning drink, and it can be made within 25 minutes.

Per Serving:

Fat: 2g | Saturated fat: 0.4g
Protein: 3g | Fiber: 1g | Sodium: 103mg

Tip:

Store in an airtight plastic wrap until you're ready to serve.

Ingredients:

- 1-1/2 cups of all-purpose flour
- 1/4 cup of egg substitute
- 1 tablespoon of sugar
- 1/4 teaspoon of ground nutmeg
- 1/2 teaspoon of ground cinnamon
- cooking spray
- 1/4 cup of dried cranberries, raisins, or currants
- 2 tablespoons of brandy or orange juice
- 1 cup of rolled oats (or quick oats)
- 3 tablespoons of reduced-fat margarine, melted
- 2-1/2 teaspoons of baking powder
- 3/4 cups skim milk

Direction:

1. Preheat oven to 400 degrees F.
2. Use cooking spray to spray a nonstick cookie sheet.
3. Place the raisins, cranberries, or currants in a small bowl with the orange juice or brandy. Allow macerating for about 15 minutes. Drain and set aside, discarding any excess orange juice or brandy.
4. Combine the rest of the ingredients in a large bowl, mixing lightly until just moistened - make sure you don't over mix it.
5. Flour your hands, and form dough into two 8-inch circles for about half-inch thick.
6. Place on prepared cookie sheet for about 4-inches apart.
7. Dip a sharp knife into flour. Cut each round into 8 pie-shaped wedges.
8. Separate the scones about half an inch from each other.
9. Bake until nicely browned, for about 12 to 15 minutes.
10. Cool on a rack and store in an airtight plastic wrap until ready to serve.
11. Enjoy.

Vegetable
Recipes

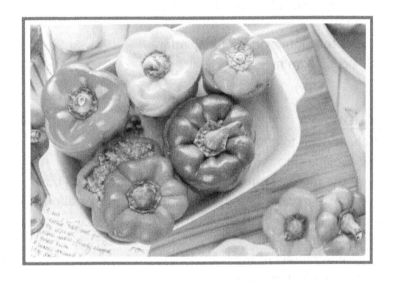

Stir-Fry Chicken Veggie

Cook Time:
1 hour

Prep Time:
15 minutes

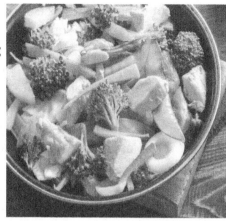

Serving Size
1

Calories per serving:
220kcal

Carbs per serving:
11g

Eating for overall diabetes prevention and good health just got a whole lot easier with this family-pleasing recipe for Stir-Fry Veggie chicken. Inactivity, obesity, a low fiber diet, and a high intake of sugar-sweetened beverages are common risk factors for diabetes, so you need this recipe to get a solution to the health problem.

Per Serving:

Fat: 9g | Saturated fat: 1.5g
Protein: 26g | Fiber: 3g |
Sodium: 380mg | Sugar: 3g

Tip:

Serve this veggie with brown rice.

Ingredients:

- 2 carrots, cut into thin rounds (about 1 cup)
- 2 cups of bite-size broccoli florets (from 1 small bunch)
- 1 medium zucchini, cut in half lengthwise and then cut into 1/4-inch-thick half-moons (about 2 cups)
- 4 garlic cloves, minced
- 2 tablespoons of reduced-sodium soy sauce, divided
- 1 tablespoon of minced fresh ginger
- Juice of 1 lime, divided
- 2 teaspoons of sesame oil, divided
- 1 pound of skinless, boneless chicken breast, cut into bite-size pieces
- 1 tablespoon of expeller pressed canola oil
- 2 green onions cut into 1/4-inch pieces (white and green parts)
- 1 jalapeño pepper, seeded and minced
- 1/4 cup of sliced fresh basil
- 1/4 cup of chopped fresh cilantro
- Brown rice, optional

Direction:

1) Place the ginger, 1 tablespoon of soy sauce, juice of half a lime, and 1 teaspoon of the sesame oil in a bowl.
2) Add the chicken pieces, seal the bag, and refrigerate for about 24 hours.
3) Heat the oil in a large nonstick skillet when ready to stir fry over medium-high heat.
4) Add the chicken and the marinade. Stir fry for about a minute.
5) Add the broccoli, carrots, green onions, garlic, and jalapeno pepper, then stir until the chicken is done and the vegetables are crisp-tender, for about 7 more minutes.
6) Stir in the rest of the soy sauce, juice, and sesame oil.
7) Stir in basil and cilantro just before serving.
8) Serve with brown rice as desired, and enjoy.

Roasted Asparagus With Bacon

Cook Time:
20 minutes

Prep Time:
5 minutes

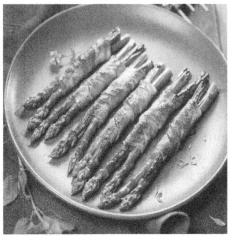

Serving Size
1

Calories per serving:
140kcal

Carbs per serving:
4g

This Roasted Asparagus with Bacon is dedicated to anyone out there who is convinced that they don't like Asparagus. The trick about them is to roast them in the oven at a high temperature that they get golden, caramelized, tender on the inside and crispy on the outside.

Per Serving:

Fat: 11g | Saturated fat: 2g
Protein: 8g | Fiber: 2g | Sodium: 370mg | Sugar: 2g

Tip:

Roasted and crisp asparagus with turkey bacon creates an irresistible side dish for Easter, or anytime.

Ingredients:

- 2 pounds of fresh asparagus, trimmed
- 1 (12-ounces) package of Jennie-O Turkey Bacon, chopped
- 2 tablespoons of olive oil

Direction:

1) Heat oven to 425 degrees F.
2) On a large rimmed baking sheet, place the asparagus.
3) Toss asparagus with turkey bacon and olive oil.
4) Spread them in a single layer.
5) Roast until asparagus is crisp-tender, for about 20 minutes.
6) Serve and enjoy.

Colorful Stuffed Peppers

Cook Time:
30 minutes

Prep Time:
5 minutes

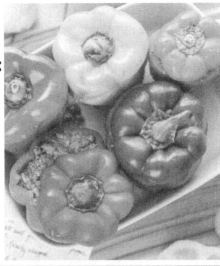

Serving Size
1

Calories per serving:
160kcal

Carbs per serving:
14g

This Colorful Turkey Stuffed Peppers recipe is for you if you're craving stuffed peppers. Extra low-fat Cheddar cheese and lean ground turkey breast make this dish irresistible.

Per Serving:

Fat: 2.5g | **Saturated fat: 1g**
Protein: 20g | Fiber: 3g |
Sodium: 210mg | Sugar: 5g

Tip:

Always cook your turkey to an internal temperature of 165 degrees F, and learn how to safely handle it.

Ingredients:

- 2 bell peppers, preferably a mix of green, yellow, or red
- 1/4 teaspoon of freshly ground black pepper
- 1 (14-1/2-ounces) can of low-sodium diced tomatoes or seasoned diced tomatoes, drained
- 1/2 cup of cooked white or brown rice
- 3/4 cup of shredded low-fat Cheddar cheese, divided
- 1/2 (16-ounce) package of Jennie-O Extra Lean Ground Turkey Breast
- 1/4 cup of chopped onion
- 2 cloves garlic, minced
- 1 tablespoon of fresh basil or 1 teaspoon of dried basil leaves
- 1/4 teaspoon of salt, if desired
- paprika, if desired
- fresh parsley, if desired

Direction:

1. Preheat the oven to 375 degrees F. Cut bell peppers lengthwise through stems. This will keep stem halves intact to hold the stuffing. Discard veins and seeds. In boiling salted water, cook peppers until crisp-tender, for about 5 minutes. Drain and place the pepper in ice water immediately to stop the cooking process. Drain peppers well, then place cut side up in 8 x 8 -inch baking dish. Cook ground turkey as specified on the package. Always cook till done when the thermometer reads 165 degrees F.

2. Add garlic, onion, salt, basil, tomatoes, ground pepper, and rice; continue to cook until heated through and most the juices have reduced, for about 5 minutes. Remove meat mixture from heat. Stir in 1/2 cup of cheese. Mound heaping half cup of mixture into each pepper half. Bake until filling is hot and peppers are tender, for about 20 minutes. Remove peppers from the oven, and sprinkle the rest of the cup cheese on top of peppers. Sprinkle with parsley and paprika, if you want. Serve and enjoy.

Tomato With Roasted Brussels Sprouts

Cook Time:
20 minutes

Prep Time:
5 minutes

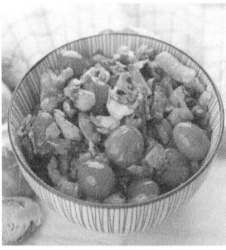

Serving Size
1

Calories per serving:
75kcal

Carbs per serving:
7g

This recipe is an oven prepared side dish recipe packed with a combination of Brussels sprouts, fire-roasted diced tomatoes, and seasonings for great flavor. It's simple, fast and very delicious.
I hope you enjoy it.

Per Serving:

Fat: 5g | Saturated fat: 0g
Protein: 2g | Fiber: 2g | Sodium: 217.6mg | Sugar: 2g

Tip:

You can assemble this dish in the morning, and place them in the refrigerator, so all you have to do is slide them in the oven at dinner. Enjoy.

Ingredients:

- 2 tablespoons of pure canola oil
- 1/4 teaspoon of garlic powder
- 1/4 teaspoon of salt
- 1 pound of small fresh Brussels sprouts, trimmed and cut in half lengthwise
- 1 can (14.5 ounces) of Hunt's Fire Roasted Diced Tomatoes, drained
- 1/8 teaspoon of ground black pepper

Direction:

1. Heat oven to 425 degrees F.
2. Toss together Brussels sprouts, oil, drained tomatoes, salt, garlic powder, and pepper in a large bowl.
3. Spread the mixture in a single layer on a large shallow baking pan.
4. Bake until Brussels sprouts are browned and tender, for about 20 minutes, stirring once halfway through.
5. Serve and enjoy.

Fish & Seafood
Recipes

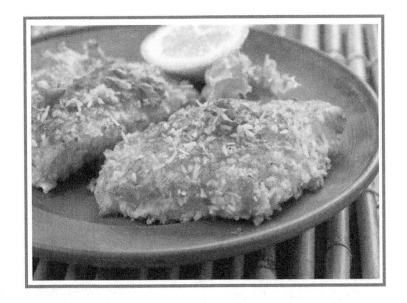

Montreal Style Salmon

Cook Time:
0 minutes

Prep Time:
15 minutes

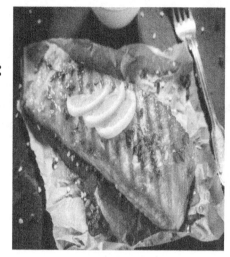

Serving Size
1

Calories per serving:
168kcal

Carbs per serving:
0g

This kind of diabetic seafood recipe provides delicious flavor for salmon on the grill. The dill weed and lemon peel are great ingredients in this recipe. I hope you enjoy it.

Per Serving:

Fat: 8g | Saturated fat: 0g
Protein: 24g | Fiber: 0g |
Sodium: 174mg

Tip:

Make sure you don't turn the salmon when using your fork.

Ingredients:

- 1/2 teaspoon of grated lemon peel
- 1/8 teaspoon of McCormick Dill Weed
- 1/2 teaspoons of McCormick Grill Mates Montreal Steak Seasoning
- 1/2 pounds of salmon fillets (swordfish or mahi-mahi can also be used)

Direction:

1. Mix steak seasoning, dill weed, and lemon peel in a small bowl.
2. Rub mixture over salmon and let it stand for about 5 minutes.
3. Grill the salmon, skin side down, over medium heat until fish flakes easily with a fork, for about 10 minutes. Make sure you don't turn the salmon.
4. Serve immediately and enjoy it.

Cracker Crusted Cod

Cook Time:
0 minute

Prep Time:
25 minutes

Serving Size
1

Calories per serving:
230kcal

Carbs per serving:
9g

This great Diabetic Crusted Cod dish can be on your dinner table in just 25 minutes. It's an excellent recipe for people that want to improve their heart health and reduce their fat intake. So if you're part of these people, do not hesitate to give it a try today. Enjoy!

Per Serving:

Fat: 12g | Saturated fat: 1.5g
Protein: 23g | Fiber: 0g |
Sodium: 300mg | Sugar: 5g

Tip:

The Crusted Cod can be in your dinner in 25 minutes. You can use breadcrumbs or panko, if you don't have crackers.

Ingredients:

- 1/4 teaspoon of salt
- 1/8 teaspoon of pepper
- 1/4 cup of fat-free (skim) milk
- 2 tablespoons of canola oil
- 1 pound of tilapia, cod, haddock, or other medium-firm fish fillets, about 3/4 inch thick
- 1/2 cup of graham cracker crumbs (about 8 squares)
- 1 teaspoon of grated lemon peel
- 2 tablespoons of chopped toasted pecans

Direction:

1. Place the oven rack to a position slightly just above the middle of the oven.
2. Heat the oven to 500 degrees F.
3. Cut the fish files crosswise into 2-inch wide pieces.
4. Mix cracker crumbs, salt, lemon peel, and pepper in a shallow dish.
5. Place milk in another shallow dish.
6. Dip fish into milk, then coat with the cracker mixture.
7. Place in the ungreased 13x9 inch pan.
8. Drizzle oil over the fish. Sprinkle with pecans.
9. Bake until the fish flakes easily with a fork, for about 10 minutes.
10. Toasting nuts adds a lot of great flavors.
11. To toast nuts bake uncovered in an ungreased shallow pan, for about 10 minutes, at 350 degrees F, occasionally stirring, until light brown.
12. Serve and enjoy.

Salmon Chowder

Cook Time:
20 minutes

Prep Time:
10 minutes

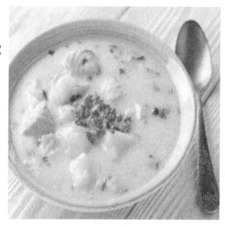

Serving Size
1
**Calories
per serving:**
280kcal
**Carbs
per serving:**
27g

This is a quick, rich, and comforting recipe

Per Serving:

Fat: 11g | Saturated fat: 2g
Protein: 18g | Fiber: 4g |
Sodium: 280mg

Tip:

You can garnish your
chowder with chopped
chives if you want.

Ingredients:

- 1/2 cup of cannellini beans, rinsed and drained
- 1/4 teaspoon of mustard powder
- 1 large garlic clove, finely chopped
- 2 teaspoons of fresh lemon juice
- 3/4 pound of skinless salmon filet, cut into 1-inch cubes
- 1 (8 ounces) bottle of clam juice
- 1/2 cup of nonfat evaporated milk
- Salt and freshly ground black pepper, to taste
- 4 teaspoons of chopped chives
- 2 tablespoons of light olive oil
- 1 onion, cut into 1/2-inch cubes
- 1 large yellow potato, peeled and diced
- 1 cup of frozen baby lima beans
- 2/3 cup of frozen yellow corn kernels

Direction:

1) In a small food processor, combine the mustard powder, beans, lemon juice, and garlic. Puree just until smooth, stopping as needed to scrape down the bowl.
2) Drizzle in the oil with the motor running. The result will look like a velvety mayonnaise; set this bean puree aside.
3) Combine potatoes, onion, and 1 1/4 cups of water in a large deep saucepan. Cover and set the pot over medium-high heat.
4) Reduce the heat to medium when the water boils for about 7 minutes. Add the corn and lima beans; cook, covered, until the potatoes are tender, for about 3 minutes longer.
5) Add the calm juice, fish, bean puree, and 1/2 cup of water.
6) Mix until the bean puree dissolves.
7) Cook over medium heat, uncovered, until fish flakes easily and opaque in the center, for about 10 minutes.
8) Take the saucepan off the heat. Stir in the milk. Then season the chowder to taste with pepper and salt.
9) Divide the soup among 4 wide, shallow bowls, and garnish with chopped chives. Serve and enjoy.

Pork & Beef
Recipes

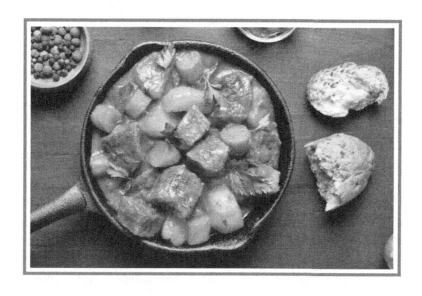

Lime Pork Tenderloin

Cook Time:
1 hour

Prep Time:
15 minutes

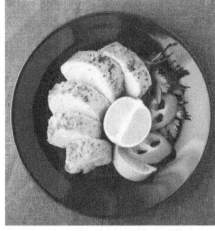

Serving Size
1

Calories per serving:
185kcal

Carbs per serving:
2g

Lime Pork Tenderloin is such an easy dinner dish suitable for you. It's ideal for weeknight dinners since it's quick-cooking and lends itself to several cooking methods. Enjoy this wonderful dish, and stay happy!

Per Serving:

Fat: 8g | Saturated fat: 2g
Protein: 24g | Fiber: 0g |
Sodium: 90mg | Sugar: 0g

Tip:

Before serving, garnish with apple slices. Then drizzle with the remaining juice from the pan.

Ingredients:

- 4 large cloves garlic, minced
- 1/2 teaspoon of chili powder, or to taste
- Salt and freshly ground pepper, to taste
- 1-1/2 pound of pork tenderloin
- 3 tablespoons of fresh lime juice
- 2 tablespoons of extra virgin olive oil, divided
- 1 teaspoon of unsulphured blackstrap molasses
- 1 tea low-sodium soy sauce
- 1 small red apple, optional for garnish

Direction:

1. Preheat oven to 375 degrees.
2. Combine lime juice, garlic, molasses, 1 tablespoon of oil, chili powder, soy sauce, pepper, and salt in a large mixing bowl.
3. Place tenderloin in a bowl, turning to coat thoroughly with marinade.
4. Heat large ovenproof pan over high heat.
5. Add the rest of the oil. Use tongs to place meat in the skillet when oil is hot, being careful to avoid splatter. Turn tenderloin for even searing to seal in juices; do this every 2 to 3 minutes.
6. Remove the pan from the burner, and pour the rest of the marinade over the meat. Brush to coat well and add 3 tablespoons of water to the skillet's bottom, not on tenderloin.
7. Place pan in the oven. Cook approx until a meat thermometer inserted into the center reads 145 degrees for about 30 minutes. Remove skillet from the oven and allow tenderloin to rest before slicing, for about 5 minutes.
8. For garnish, cut the apple in thin slices, if using.
9. Cut tenderloin diagonally in 1/4-1/2 inch slices.
10. Arrange slices on a plate. Garnish with apple slices. Then drizzle with the remaining juice from the pan.
11. Serve and enjoy.

Grilled Pork Tenderloin

Cook Time:
50 minutes

Prep Time:
30 minutes

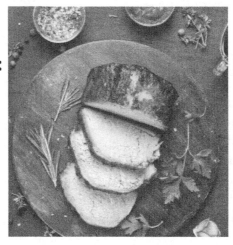

Serving Size
1

Calories per serving:
238.9kcal

Carbs per serving:
21.5g

For a quick and elegant dinner, this pork recipe is the kind of recipe you should go for. Add a grill roasted potatoes and green salad together to get the final result. I have paired the meat with a zesty sweet and sour rhubarb chutney for a classic flavor combo.
Enjoy!

Per Serving:

Fat: 1.3g | **Saturated fat:** 1.3g
Protein: 24.7g | **Fiber:** 1.5g |
Sodium: 330.5mg | **Calcium:**
64.9mg | **Potassium:** 669.7mg |
Sugar: 17.8g

Tip:

If you want to make ahead, refrigerate chutney for up to 3 days.

Ingredients:

- 1 tablespoon of rice vinegar
- 3 tablespoons of honey
- 1 tablespoon of brown sugar
- 1/2 teaspoon of granulate garlic
- 1/4 teaspoon of smoked salt
- 1 tablespoon of extra-virgin olive oil
- 1/2 cup of finely diced yellow onion
- 1/4 teaspoon of kosher salt
- 1 clove garlic, minced
- 2 teaspoons of grated fresh ginger
- 2 cups of thinly sliced rhubarb, fresh or frozen (thawed)
- 1 pound of pork tenderloin, trimmed

Direction:

1) Preheat grill to medium. In a medium saucepan, heat oil over medium heat, and add kosher salt and onion.
2) Cook, occasionally stirring, for about 3 minutes, until soft but not brown. Add minced ginger and garlic; cook, occasionally stirring, for about a minute.
3) Add rhubarb and cook, stirring occasionally, for about 5 minutes until it is mostly broken down.
4) Stir in vinegar, scraping up any browned bits.
5) Add honey. Reduce heat to maintain a simmer.
6) Cook, occasionally stirring, for about 2 to 6 minutes, until the chutney is thickened. Remove from heat. Cover to keep warm.
7) Combine granulated garlic, brown sugar, and smoked salt in a small bowl. Sprinkle evenly over pork.
8) Oil the grill rack and grill the pork until an instant-read thermometer inserted into the thickest part reads 145 degrees, occasionally turning, for about 12 minutes.
9) Transfer to a clean cutting board. Let it rest for about 5 minutes. Slice the pork, then serve with the rhubarb chutney.
10) Enjoy.

Beef Goulash

Cook Time:
2 hours

Prep Time:
15 minutes

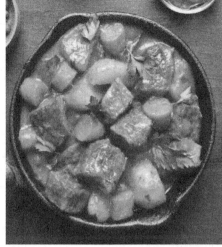

Serving Size
1

**Calories
per serving:**
370kcal

**Carbs
per serving:**
39.6g

This Beef Goulash is an excellent dish for your immune system, skin,
brain, and eyesight. I hope you enjoy it.

Per Serving:

Fat: 8.7g | **Saturated fat:** 2.8g
Protein: 32.1g | **Fiber:** 6.2g |
Sugar: 12.1g

Tip:

You could use lamb or pork in this recipe instead of beef. You can also use tofu in place of beef to make a vegetarian version.

Ingredients:

- 1 clove garlic, crushed
- 1 teaspoon of paprika
- 1 x 200grams can of chopped tomatoes
- 1 tablespoon of tomato puree
- 250grams of lean braising steak, cubed
- 250grams of potatoes
- 2 teaspoons of seasoned flour
- 1 teaspoon of oil
- 1 onion, chopped
- half red pepper, chopped
- 150ml (quarter pint) of beef stock

Direction:

1. Preheat the oven to 180 degrees C.
2. Toss the steak in the seasoned flour.
3. In a flameproof casserole dish, heat the oil and add the steak. Then fry until browned all over, for about 2 to 3 minutes.
4. Add the rest of the ingredients, bring to the boil, then cover and place in the oven.
5. Cook until the meat is tender, for about 2 hours.
6. Serve with plenty of vegetables.
7. Enjoy.

Drinks
Recipes

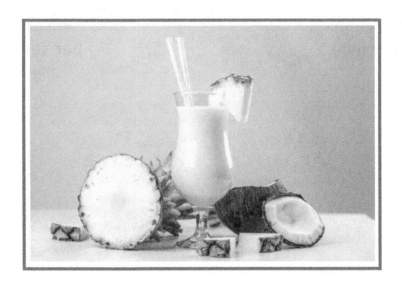

No-Sugar Pina Colada

Cook Time:
0 minute

Prep Time:
15 minutes

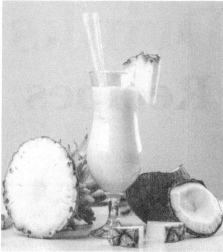

Serving Size
1
**Calories
per serving:**
210kcal
**Carbs
per serving:**
25g

There are several levels to achieve the same level of sweetness without adding sugar. So, this recipe gives answers to your problems. This version of Pina Colada is the best you'll ever try. Enjoy!

Per Serving:

Fat: 3g | Saturated fat: 2.5g
Protein: 1g | Fiber: 2g | Sodium:
10mg | Sugar: 17g

Tip:

Before serving, garnish with a slice of pineapple.

Ingredients:

- 3 fluid ounces of white rum
- 1/3 cup of lite coconut milk
- A handful of ice cubes
- 1/4 cup of cold water
- 2 packets of Splenda Naturals Stevia Sweetener
- 12 ounces of frozen pineapple chunks

Direction:

1) Add all the ingredients in a blender.
2) Pulse until smooth, stopping, then scraping down the sides if you want.
3) Pour in your glass cup.
4) Garnish with a slice of fresh pineapple.
5) Serve immediately and enjoy it.

Strawberry Smoothie

Cook Time:

0 minute

Prep Time:

5 minutes

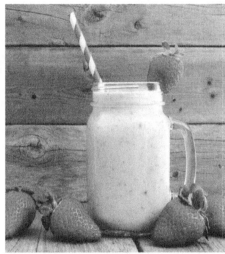

Serving Size

1

Calories per serving:

80kcal

Carbs per serving:

16g

This recipe is so good that you'll think you're drinking a milkshake. What makes me love this Strawberry smoothie is the non-fat plain yogurt added. The combination of yogurt and strawberries calls my attention. I prepared it, and they come out great!

Per Serving:

Fat: 0g | Saturated fat: 0g
Protein: 5g | Fiber: 0g | Sodium: 60mg

Tip:

This is a recipe made quickly and easily in a blender.

Ingredients:

- 6 tablespoons of Equal Spoonful or Granulated
- 3 cups of frozen unsweetened whole strawberries
- 1 cup of ice cubes
- 1 cup of nonfat plain yogurt
- 1/4 cup of fat-free milk
- 9 packets Equal sweetener

Direction:

1. Combine milk, yogurt, and Equal in a blender or a food processor, then cover.
2. Add the berries with the blender running, a few at a time, through an opening in the lid.
3. Process until smooth.
4. Add the ice cubes, one at a time, through the lid opening, blending just until slushy, and pouring into glasses.
5. Serve immediately and enjoy it.

Frozen Coffee Whip

Cook Time:
0 minute

Prep Time:
5 minutes

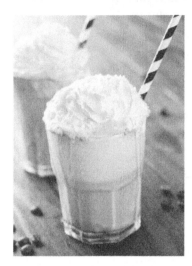

Serving Size
1

**Calories
per serving:**
50kcal

**Carbs
per serving:**
8g

The result of this Frozen Coffee Whip is a super creamy and rich iced coffee drink that is so easy and fun to make at home. Do not forget to add the vanilla to this drink because it gives it a nice flavor! Get to your kitchen now and make yours!

Per Serving:

Fat: 2g | **Saturated fat:** 1.5g
Protein: 1g | **Fiber:** 0g | **Sodium:**
40mg | **Sugar:** 3g

Tip:

Serve with Cool Whip
Sugar-Free Topping, and
enjoy your coffee!

Ingredients:

- 2 tablespoons of fat-free half-and-half
- 2 teaspoons of Splenda no Calorie sweetener, Granulated
- 1/4 teaspoon of vanilla
- 1 cup of ice cubes
- 3 tablespoons of thawed cool whip sugar-free whipped topping, divided
- 1/4 cup of brewed strong maxwell house Italian espresso roast coffee, cooled

Direction:

1. Reserve 1 tablespoon of cool whip.
2. Blend the rest of the cool whip with all the remaining ingredients except ice in a blender, just until well blended.
3. Add ice and blend until smooth and thickened at high speed.
4. Serve topped with the rest of the cool whip.
5. Enjoy!

Conclusion

Congratulations on making it to the end of this journey with me. Living with diabetes is difficult; it's an unfortunate hand many of us are dealt. But, with the right diet and lifestyle, we can make life much easier and enjoyable for ourselves.

Going forward, I wish you the best of luck. You've taken the first big step towards a better and happier you by finishing this book. I can only hope it helps you to reach whatever goals you have set for yourself, whether that be weight loss or just general healthier eating.

Please remember that as beneficial as dieting and healthy eating is, it isn't a cure and it won't fix your diabetes. If you have any serious medical conditions or suspect you may have some, please see a registered health care professional.

Thank you for reading, and good luck!

References

Bandurski, K. (2019, July 18). *35 Diabetic-Friendly Recipes to Pack for Lunch*. Taste of Home. https://www.tasteofhome.com/collection/diabetic-lunch-recipes/

Bandurski, K. (2020, August 30). *50 Chicken Recipes for People With Diabetes*. Taste of Home. https://www.tasteofhome.com/collection/diabetic-chicken-recipes/

Centers for Disease Control and Prevention. (2016). *New CDC report: More than 100 million Americans have diabetes or prediabetes*. https://www.cdc.gov/media/releases/2017/p0718-diabetes-report.html

Centers for Disease Control and Prevention. (2019). *Type 2 Diabetes*. https://www.cdc.gov/diabetes/basics/type2.html

Cohen, L. (2018, February 7). *55 Quick and Easy Healthy Breakfasts for Your Busiest Mornings*. Good Housekeeping. https://www.goodhousekeeping.com/food-recipes/easy/g871/quick-breakfasts/

Curry, K. (2015, February 7). *Hacking Meal Prep: Tips, Tricks & Recipes!* Fit Men Cook. https://fitmencook.com/hacking-meal-prep-tips-tricks-recipes/

Davis, S. (n.d.). *Eating Well With Type 2 Diabetes*. WebMD. https://www.webmd.com/diabetes/features/eating-well-type-2-diabetes

Diabetes UK. (2017). *10 Tips for Healthy Eating With Diabetes*. https://www.diabetes.org.uk/guide-to-diabetes/enjoy-food/eating-with-diabetes/10-ways-to-eat-well-with-diabetes

Diabetes.co.uk. (2019a). *Cataracts and Diabetes - Causes of Cataracts, Symptoms & Treatment*. https://www.diabetes.co.uk/diabetes-complications/cataracts.html

Diabetes.co.uk. (2019). *Causes of Diabetes - What Causes Diabetes?* https://www.diabetes.co.uk/diabetes-causes.html

Diimig, C. (n.d.). *5-Day Diabetes Meal Plan for Weight Loss*. Eating Well. http://www.eatingwell.com/article/291368/5-day-diabetes-meal-plan-for-weight-loss/

Dresden, D. (2019, April 23). *Lunch ideas for type 2 diabetes: Ingredients, recipes, and eating out.* Medical News Today. https://www.medicalnewstoday.com/articles/317154#tips

EatingWell.com. (2020, August 9). *The Best 30-Day Diabetes Diet Plan.* http://www.eatingwell.com/gallery/12933/the-best-30-day-diabetes-diet-plan/?

Elliott, B. (2018, January 14). *The 21 Best Snack Ideas If You Have Diabetes.* Healthline. https://www.healthline.com/nutrition/best-snacks-for-diabetes#section5

Hoskins, M. (2020, May 1). *Neuropathy: Dealing with Dreaded Diabetes Nerve Pain.* Healthline. https://www.healthline.com/diabetesmine/neuropathy-and-type1-diabetes#:~:text=Neuropathy%20is%20one%20of%20othe

Kivi, R., & Boskey, E. (2020, June 17). *Type 1 Diabetes: Symptoms, Treatment, Causes, and Vs. Type 2.* Healthline. https://www.healthline.com/health/type-1-diabetes-causes-symtoms-treatments#treatment

Manfred, E. (2020, June 5). *All About the Hemoglobin A1c Test.* Healthline. https://www.healthline.com/health/type-2-diabetes/ac1-test#how-it-works

Mealplanmagic.com. (2018, May 7). *The Ultimate Guide to Meal Prep Storage and How to Keep Your Meals Fresh.* https://www.mealplanmagic.com/blogs/meal-planning/the-ultimate-guide-to-meal-preparation#3

Norman, J. (2019). *Treatment of Diabetes: The Diabetic Diet.* EndocrineWeb. https://www.endocrineweb.com/conditions/diabetes/treatment-diabetes

Oerum, C. (2017, November 5). *7-Day Diabetes Meal Plan (With Printable Grocery List).* Diabetes Strong. https://diabetesstrong.com/my-fit-diabetic-meal-plan/

Petre, A. (2018, September 30). *How to Meal Prep — A Beginner's Guide.* Healthline. https://www.healthline.com/nutrition/how-to-meal-prep#9

Pietrangelo, A. (2014, July 24). *Understanding Type 2 Diabetes.* Healthline. https://www.healthline.com/health/type-2-diabetes#diet

Racette Parulski, E. (2019, September 19). *60 Incredibly Delicious Diabetic-Friendly Dinners.* Taste of Home.

https://www.tasteofhome.com/collection/delicious-diabetic
-friendly-dinner-recipes/

Seaver, V. (2019, February 23). *The Best 7-Day Diabetes Meal Plan.*
EatingWell.
http://www.eatingwell.com/article/290459/the-best-7-day-
diabetes-meal-plan/

Sissons, B. (2019, February 12). *10 best foods for diabetes: What to
eat and avoid.* Medical News Today.
https://www.medicalnewstoday.com/articles/324416#probi
otic-yogurt

Spritzler, F. (2017a, January 29). *13 Ways to Prevent Type 2
Diabetes.* Healthline.
https://www.healthline.com/nutrition/prevent-diabetes#16

Spritzler, F. (2017b, February 6). *11 Foods to Avoid with Type 2
Diabetes.* Healthline.
https://www.healthline.com/nutrition/foods-to-avoid-with-
diabetes#section5

Spritzler, F. (2017c, June 3). *The 16 Best Foods to Control Diabetes.*
Healthline.
https://www.healthline.com/nutrition/16-best-foods-for-di
abetics#section17

Watson, S. (2018, October 4). *Everything You Need to Know About
Diabetes.* Healthline.
https://www.healthline.com/health/diabetes#symptoms

WebMD.com. (2007). *Causes of Type 2 Diabetes.* .
https://www.webmd.com/diabetes/diabetes-causes

WebMD.com. (2008, July 30). *Best and Worst Foods for Diabetes.*
https://www.webmd.com/diabetes/diabetic-food-list-best-
worst-foods

WebMD.com. (2019, August 20). *10 Tips for Eating Well With
Diabetes.*
https://www.webmd.com/a-to-z-guides/condition-15/diabe
tes/tips-eat-well?page=2

Made in United States
North Haven, CT
24 June 2024

53993420R00157